REPRODUCTIVE AND CHILD HEALTH

Ankur Yadav

RAJAT PUBLICATIONS
New Delhi

Reproductive and Child Health
by *Ankur Yadav*

This edition is published by Rajat Publications
4740/23, Ansari Road Daryaganj,
New Delhi - 110002

ISBN: 978-81-7880-228-2

Edition 2025

Rs. 1295/-

Printed and bound in India

RAJAT
PUBLICATIONS

4740/23, Ansari Road, Daryaganj,
New Delhi- 110002 (India)
Tel:- +91-11-23267924
Mob:- +91-9811484973, +91-9811105389
E-mail: rajat_publication@yahoo.com

Dedicated

to

My Parents

Shri Radhe Shyam Yadav

&

Smt. Devatmja Yadav

Preface

Tribal population of India lives in widely varying ecological and geoclimatic condition in different concentration throughout the country. They are characterized by their distinct socio-cultural and biological set-up. The health status of these tribal population groups is as such a function of the interaction between their socio-cultural and socio-biological practices, genetic attributes and the environmental condition.

Madhya Pradesh a hub having a large concentration of tribal population. Tribal groups inhabiting various interior and remote region, which lack even elementary healthcare facilities, are exposed to environmental stress and strain. Due to hostile environmental conditions, they suffer from specific types of health problems. In view of the National Health Care Policy (NHCP) and National commitment to achieve "Health for all by A.D. 2000" through primary healthcare approach, the studies on scheduled tribes / scheduled castes and minority communities become priority groups for providing ensuring better healthcare services.

A critical review clearly indicate that hardly and holistic study carried out among the tribal population on the Reproductive and Child Health profile especially in Madhya Pradesh tribal groups. Such data are important for planning of effective need based, area and group specific health care strategies in these groups, where the available reports revealed that they tend to under utilise the available health care facilities. So each tribe has to be studied carefully so as to develop effective health care measures. Keeping this in view embodied study has been carried among the Raj Gonds of Sagar District, Madhya Pradesh.

I am deeply beholden to my mentor Dr. K.K.N. Sharma, Lecturer, Department of Anthropology, Dr. H.S. Gour University, who introduced me to this fascinating and interesting field of tribal research. His valuable guidance and encouragement cannot be overlooked in my career.

I express my gretefulness to Dr. D. Sukhla (Reader), Department of Mathematics & Statistics, Dr. H.S. Gour University, Sagar. Dr, G.D. Pandey and Mr. Anil Ghual, R.M.R.C., I.C.M.R., Jabalpur and Dr. Smt. Kalpana Sharma for all kinds of help he extended to me to make the study successful.

I am also grateful to Shri S.K. Tiwari and Shri Dwarika Sen who firstly introduced me with Raj Gonds and the people among whom, I had worked, without whose co-operation the present work would not be possible at all.

I wish to register my note of thanks to my colleagues for their sweet memories and valuable help during the course of work—Mr. Pavan & Mrs. Manju Vishwakarma, Miss Meenakshi Yadav, Miss Swati Patni, Miss Rosy Anita Kerkatta, Miss Chetana Khare, Mr. Narendra Upadhyaya, Mr. Satyam Dave, Mr. Vinod Agnihotri and Mr. Bahadur Singh Tomar, Mr. Abhishek Yadav, Mr. Narendra Singh Thakur and Mr. Mahesh Thakur. I offer my personal thanks to my senior Dr. Dipak Adak.

No word can adequately express my debt of gratitude to my parents who have been always a perennial source of energy for me and my academic pursuit and life.

Ankur Yadav

CONTENTS

The scheduled tribes in our country inhabit in low economic status, who do not have adequate access to affordable health care services. They remain under-served in the coverage of reproductive and child health services. These communities need special attention of basis health and reproductive and child health services (National Population Policy, 2000). Thus, there is an urgent need to re-organise and re-structure the development programme in view of their health need, which have to be identified, mainly with reference to their health and hygienic background, socio-cultural practices and traditional health care system.

It has been estimated by the World Health Organisation (2000) that more than 514,000 women die each year from complications of pregnancy and childbirth (i.e., one per minute) and 99 per cent of these maternal deaths occur in developing countries. Perhaps 15 times as many suffer injury or infection. Each year more than 50 million pregnancy-related complications lead to long-term illness and disability. With 36.1 million people now living with HIV/AIDS and 5.3 million new infections in 2000, urgency cannot be overstated. One half of all people who become infected with HIV are under the age of 25. 78,000 women die each year from unsafe abortion, almost all in developing countries. The United Nations has called upon countries to reduce unwanted pregnancies and deal with the health impact of unsafe abortion as a major public-health concern. 350 million couples do not have access to a choice of safe and affordable contraceptive methods. Surveys from more than 60 developing countries indicate that more than 100 million women who are not currently using a contraceptive method want to delay the birth of their next child or to stop having children.

At least one in every three women has been beaten,

coerced into sex or abused—most often by someone she knows. Each year 2 million girls are at risk of female genital mutilation. As many as 5,000 women and girls are killed each year in so-called "honour killings". Refugees, internally displaced persons and others caught in situations of conflict or emergency face particular challenges to their reproductive rights, from family planning needs to treatment and counselling in cases of sexual violence and rape (Fourth World Conference on Women in Beijing in 1995).

India alone loses more than 1,00,000 women every year in this pursuit (WHO, 1991). Maternal mortality ratio has been estimated to be 555 per 1,00,000 live births (Bhatt, *et al.* 1992), which is fifty times higher than that in neighbouring Srilanka (UNICEF, 1991, Ascadi and Ascadi, 1990). It has been estimated that India accounts for at least 27 % of all maternal deaths in the world (Ranjan, 1998). In Madhya Pradesh, maternal deaths in 1993, accounted for more than 4 % of the total female deaths and almost on fifth of the total female deaths were in the child bearing years (Govt. of M.P., 1993). UNICEF (1998) has estimated a maternal mortality ratio of 738 deaths per 100,000 live births on the basis of empirical association that exists between mortality ratio and infant mortality rate.

The theme of Reproductive and Child Health (RCH) care offers a vast area of research. Many studies have been carried out so far. Most of the available studies are based on hospital data and national sample surveys. Murali and Kotaria (1980), Jha (1983) and Saksena (1988) observed that the lack of clinical attendance of pregnant mother is due to the lack of knowledge and distantly situated health centres. Khan and Rao (1989) study on Bihar exhibits that the health delivery system did not benefit the poor who are in most need study on Madras city revealed that Mother and Child Health (MCH) services are much influenced by the factors like education, occupation, income, accessibility and the like (Yesudian, 1989). Whereas Srinivasan and Sugathan's (1976) has empirical analysed in six primary health centres in rural Bangalore revealed a positive relationship between acceptance of sterilisation and type of maternal and child health care received by women. Regarding utilisation pattern of Mother and Child Health (MCH) care services, different studies showed that a considerable proportion of women did not use either Ante Natal Care (ANC) or delivery services due to ignorance, lack of cooperation among family members and rude behaviour of hospital staff (Mandakini, 1971; Kumar, 1982; Caldwell, 1986; Ravindran, 1988; Basu, 1990). Parker and Wolff (1984) and Kaul (1991) found that attitudes, beliefs and socio-economic factors had some impact on the use of health services. Regarding maternal morbidity Bhatia and Cleland (1994) BCC (1980), Datta, (1980), Knowless (1987), Randhawa and Kanwar (1990), Jacobson (1993), Bhattacharya *et al.* (1993), Ramachandran and Muthuswamy (1994) and Hutter (1994) conducted their studies in different population of India. Sharma and Sharma (1992), Pathak and Ram (1993), Maitra *et al.* (1994), Begum *et al.* (1998) have reported health profile and pregnancy complications associated with adolescent mothers in different rural setup of the country. There are numerous KAP (Knowledge, Attitude and Practices) studies available on the health status of the tribals in India's (Arora and Choudhary, 1993, Jaiswal, 1985, Jaiswal and Singh, 1989; Rajayalakshmi, 1991; Sahay, 1993; Sahay and Singh, 1995; Singh *et al.* 1987 a & b 1988, 1991 and 1996; Pandey, *et al.*, 1996; Pandey, 1999; Jain, 2000; Dwivedi, 2003; Parchure and Warvadekar, 2004).

The accessibility of health centres within a reachable distance greatly enhances the utilisation of medical facilities and family planning services (Ghosh and Mukherjee, 1989). Vijayakumar and Chhakrapani (1995), Pathak and Singh (1993), Bharati and Basu (1990) reported anemia to be one of the major causes of maternal mortality and morbidity. Various studies on the knowledge and utilisation of child immunisation revealed that education and different socio economic factor of the community has a great influence (Jorapur, 1979; Sengupta and Kumar, 1977; Shukla 1980; Caldwell, 1982; Sharma and Sharma, 1992; Premrajan and Srinivasan, 1994; Rohde, 1992). A investigation in Kerala it has been obsessed that immunisation coverage of pregnant women is satisfactory but about child it is too poor (Malhotra, 1988).

A good number of studies concerned with knowledge, awareness and utilisation of family welfare services are available which revealed that there is a gap between knowledge and actual practice of family welfare services and again knowledge is directly related with the level of literacy (Ahmed, 1973; Dutta, 1973; Siddh, 1974; Kohli and Goel, 1974; Prasad, 1977; Bhatia and Newmann, 1980; Mahadevan, 1983; Vlassoff, 1984 and Srivastava and Saksena, 1988; Zoe and Mahendra, 2001; Suman and Ansari, 2001; Paruthi and Gupta, 2001; Gupta, 2001; Chandra, 2001; Abou Zahr and Wardlaw, 2001; Agarwal, 2001; Begum and Nurul Islam, 2001; Bajpai, 2001; Yadav et al. 2002). Gulati (1971), Sebastian (1972), Alwani (1976), Bhargawa (1983), Singhal (1992), Sarker (2000), Sharma *et al.* (2002) reported that parents literacy level, status and occupation are significantly associated with immunisation coverage.

In India slums constitute the most persistent problem of urban life, the majority of urban dwellers waging a continued and increasingly desperate battle for survival. Education and health facilities take the lowest priority. Contraceptive use among slum population is influenced by the availability as-well-as a number of social, economic and cultural characteristics (Gupta, 1991; Prasad and Somayajulu, 1992). Pethe, (1962), Seetalaxmi (1969), Koteswar (1970), Devi (1972), Operations Research Group

(1974) and Purnia and Singh (1984) studies on Knowledge Attitude and Practice (KAP) has been conducted by various workers (Balakrishna, 1971; Das, 1972; Mukherjee, 1975; Srinivasan *et al.* 1976; Pandey & Tiwari, 1993).

Mamgain (1972) emphasized the role of MCH in bringing about the concept of small family norm. Kale (1966) studied in Dharwar district and found that small family norm had not reached the rural areas. Among hut dwellers in Patna, Prasad (1977) revealed that though 97% of families have the knowledge of family planning but very few did use since they feel insecure about the survivality of their children due to high child mortality. A study by Mouli and Mouli (1981) in Ramnagar Taluk of Bangalore district revealed that economic constraints necessitated people to adopt family planning Kaur and Singh (1982) found that education is the main key in acceptance of family welfare services. Shariff (1989) explains the regional variation in use of family planning is due to low female literacy and other socio-cultural backwardness. Visaria and Visaria (1990) have revealed that low utilisation of family planning services is due to non- accessibility of the contraceptive methods. Mahadevan's study (1983) on non-acceptance of family planning methods revealed that it is due to inadequate knowledge and ignorance of its importance. While Khan (1985) in their study in Uttar Pradesh found that women were keen to accept family planning but the non-availability of contraceptives is the main hindrance.

Noteworthy Contributions in the Field of Proposed Work

In recent years there has been a growing concern for women's health in developing countries, since family planning and mother and child health care survives can improve their survival and quality of life (UNICEF, 1989). In India the National Family Health Survey (NFHS, 1992-93) carried out by the Ministry of Family Welfare (MOFW) in coordination with International Institute of Population

Sciences (IIPS), Mumbai provide a complete information on implementation and effectiveness of Mother and Child Health and Family Planning Services. In 1993 the King Edward Hospital, Pune in association with Indian Council of Medical Research (ICMR) conducted an action research study for implementation of a package of interventions for improving maternal and child health services in rural areas, through training, supervision and educating the community on the need of MCH services (Ranganathan and Rao, 1993). Sengupta and Gode (1987) presented a nine years review on maternal morbidity and mortality from some North-Indian Hospitals. Anaemia is quite common in women and children in rural areas. Maternal malnutrition leads to premature deliveries, low birth weight babies and pregnancy watages. It is found that tribal women during pregnancy also engage in hard manual works, and no additional diet has been found to take by them. In most of the tribes delivery are conducted at home by elderly ladies/dais. Performance of immunisation in tribal regions was found highly inadequate. A high male gender preference among the Oraon and Munda make female children more prone to develop severe malnutrition (Singh, 1983 and Chopra, 1999). The information on incidence of reproductive was age and still birth are under estimated due to their socio-cultural constraints (Murthy and Ramesh, 1978 and Sharma, 1979). The World Health Organisation (1981) conducted a collaborative study on breast feeding in nine developing countries including India between 1975-78 and found socio-cultural factors such as education, employment, income and urban residence to be the strongest determinants of the length of breast feeding. Thimmayamma & Vidyavati (1980) and Walia *et al.,* (1974) reported that almost all mothers consider breast milk is best food for infants however, the actual practice is in sharp contrast to this belief. Ramachandran (1983) and Reddy (1995) in their studies found a negative interrelationship between breast feeding and infant morality.

A critical review of the literature clearly indicates that hardly any holistic study has been carried out on tribal groups especially in Madhya Pradesh, regarding reproductive and child health care. Therefore it is essential to find out their health problems associated with genetic and socio-cultural factors for the formulation of need based, area and group specific health care programmes. Keeping this in view, present study has been carried out in Raj Gond of Sagar district, Madhya Pradesh.

The Objectives of the Present Study

1. To investigate the maternal and child mortality and morbidity patterns and associated factors.
2. To elicit their Knowledge Attitudes and Practices (KAP) Regarding Reproductive and Child Health (RCH) problems.

2
Geographical Location and People

India

India is a land of numerous diversity from north to south and east to west. India is situated in the South Asia between latitudes 8°4' and 37°6' north, longitudes 68°7' and 97°25' east and measure about 3,214 km. from north to south between the extreme latitudes and about 2,933 km. from east to west between the extreme longitudes. It has a land frontier of about 15,200 km. The total length of the coast line is 7,516.6 km. India is bounded in north west by Pakistan and Afghanistan, China, Tibet, Bhutan and Nepal to north, Myanmar and Bangladesh to east. It covers an area of 32,87,263 sq. km. extending from the snow covered Himalayan heights to tropical rain forests of the south. The entire India can be divided into seven major physiographic regions. Northern mountains including the Himalayas and the mountains ranges in the north-east, Indo-Gangetic plain, Central Highlands, Peninsular Islands, East Coast, West Coast, Bordering Seas and Islands. The constitution of India was adapted by the constituent assembly on 26 November 1949 and came into force on January 26,1950 since than it has been amended 85 times. There are 397 articles and nine schedules, which form a comprehensive document. The union of India comprises 28 states, six union territories and one national capital territory. The population of India according to 2001 census is million and is the home of 16 per cent of world's population. It has 439.23 million males and 407.07 million females. The literacy rate in the country (excluding Jammu & Kashmir) was 52.21 per cent (64.13 per cent for males and 39.29 per cent for females). Hindus, Muslims, Christians, Sikhs, Buddhists, Jains and Parsis are the major religious communities of India. India has 18 officially recognised languages. 1971 census listed 1652 languages as mother languages spoken in India out of these 1652 languages, 33 are spoken by people numbering over a lakh. The country has an area of 752.3 lakh hectare notified as forests, 406.1 lakh hectares is classified as reserved and 215 lakh hectares as protected unclassified forest area is spread over 131.1 lakh hectares. About 19.47 per cent of the total geographical area of country is under actual forest cover. The National Wildlife Action Plan (1982) provides the framework of strategy as well as programme for conservation of wildlife. India has 80 national parks and 441 sanctuaries, which covers area of 4.15 per cent of the graphical area of the country area of the country. The major rivers of the Himalayan group are Indus, Ganges and Brahmaputra and the main rivers of the Decan are Krishna, Cauvery, Mahanadi, Narmada and Tapti.

Madhya Pradesh

The state of Madhya Pradesh is the third largest state of India, in terms of area, and the seventh largest in terms of population. It covers about 9.2 per cent of the country's total geographic area. It is unique in the sense that it has no sea and no connection with Himalayas and yet it has some extremely charming hills and mountains and has some big rivers, with an area of 308245 sq. km. having 313 development blocks, 259 tehsils, 45 districts and 9 commissionarates.

The state is located in the central part of India and, therefore, it is called as *Madhya Pradesh*. Its comprises of two words "Madhya" and "Pradesh" of Hindi language, which means "Central" and "State" respectively, so it means "Central State". In 1956, Madhya Pradesh was founded by the merger of former Madhya Pradesh, Bhopal, Vindhya Pradesh and the Central Province region of the former province of Central Prant and Berar. Now, Bhopal is the capital of the state. On 1st November, 2000 Madhya Pradesh was again divided into Madhya Pradesh and Chhattisgarh.

The state has a population of 6,03,85,118 people comp arises of 31,457 thousand male and 28,928 thousand females according to the 2001 census. Which is 5.88% of the India There are 46 scheduled tribes comprising 161 tribal sub-groups in the state. Three largest tribal groups of the state are the Gonds (44.60 per cent), Bhil and Bhilala (20.84 per cent), and Kanwar (4.67 per cent). The primitive tribal groups numbering three, viz. Baiga, Bharia, and Sahariya.

Madhya Pradesh is rich in wild life, Tigers are found in many parts of the state. There are as many as 9 national parks and 22 sanctuaries in the state. The tiger, leopard, deer, chittal, sambhar, barasingha, neelgai, and gour are the protected animals. It has many national parks and wildlife sanctuaries, such as, Kanha National Park and Shivpuri National Park.

An area of about 1.2 million hectares of land in the state is under-forest. Madhya Pradesh is one of the most forested state of India. Teak, sal, bamboo and tendu leaves are the important forest products of the state.

Madhya Pradesh is predominantly agriculture-based state and about 80 per cent of population depends on agriculture for their livelihood. Nearly, 44 per cent of available land is used for cultivation and only about 18 per cent of the cultivated land is being irrigated.

Madhya Pradesh is one of the mineral important state of India. It has depositions of various minerals, *viz.* coal, iron, bauxite, limestone and manganese. The Panna region is famous for the production of diamonds and other precious stones like neelam, panna etc.

The entire state can be divided into ten agro-climatic regions, i.e.

1. Northern hill plateau, 2. Kymore plateau, 3. Satpura hills, 4. Vindhyan hills, 5. Central Narmada valley, 6. Gird region, 7. Satpura plateau, 8. Malwa plateau, 9. Nimar plateau, 10. Jhabua hills.

The literacy of the state is below the national average of 52.21 per cent. Its achievement in this area is 66.11 per cent. The fact that Madhya Pradesh has a high proportion of scheduled tribes, as much as 23 per cent would also account for the low of progress in the vital sector.

Madhya Pradesh has been part and parcel of the main current of Indian history and culture since ancient times. It was the part of Mauryan empire, based in Pataliputra (modern Patna) and the great Ashoka, Grandson of the founder of the dynasty Chandragupta Maurya in Madhya Pradesh. In 17th and 18th centuries Marathas established two major states of Indore and Gwalior in Madhya Pradesh.

There are some areas of ethnobotanical significance such as Amarkantak, Pachmarhi, Shivpuri, Chhindwara and Kanha etc. Pachmarhi is a prominent hill station of the state situated in Hoshangabad district about 40 km. away from the district headquarters.

The river 'Narmada' originates at Amarkantak and flows westward and a little distance away the "Sone" river rises to flow eastwards a kind of phenomena, which is most unusual anywhere in the world. The river Narmada has a prehistorical importance because from its bank "*Homoerectus narmadensis* " was recovered.

Some historic paintings are also found in the "Bagh Caves", 160 km. away from Indore, which resembles those at Ajanta in Maharashtra and they are believed to belong to a period between 5th and 7th centuries A.D.

Sagar District

The district Sagar lie on the hills of Vindhyan plateau. The district is surrounded by seven other districts *i.e.* Guna, Vidisha, Raisen, Damoh, Narshingpur, Chhatarpur and Lalitpur. Sagar lies between 22°10′ to 24°27′ north and 78° to 79°21' east. Its extreme length is about 169 kms from north to west and extreme breadth 120 kms, from east to west and total area of the district is about 10,252 sq km. Sagar district is divided into seven tehsils they are Sagar, Banda, Bina, Deori, Rehli, Garhakota and Khurai.

History

The records of the history of Sagar district is available from the 1022 A.D. Initially, Sagar was under the rules of "Ahir-Rajas" and their capital was the present Garphera site. Ahir-Rajas were defeated by Raja Nihal Singh in 1023 A.D. after that he and his descendents ruled in Sagar. In 1660 "Oddenshah" founded the present Sagar town. After him, his grandson Prathavipath in 1732 was defeated by Kurba Nawab. Kurba Nawab was defeated by Peshwa Bajjirav and handed this area to Govind Rao Pandit. In 1818 Bajjirav handed most of the Sagar district portions to East India Company. In 1858 British Government took the charge of whole India including Sagar from the East India Company. In 1866, British government made Sagar as a district in Madhya Prant.

Earlier Sagar was situated in the present Garphera site and that was the old Sagar, but some "Banjaras" collectively dug big lake of Sagar and then the old Sagar was shifted from Garphera site to the present site situated on the north and west bank of Sagar lake and due to the

(i) Summer

This season starts from middle of March and ends in the mid of June. Average temperature of the season is 33.3°C which varies from 17.8°C to 49.8°C.

(ii) Rainy

It Starts from June and ends in September. Monsoon brings the rain in the district. Average rainfall in the district is 1235 mm. Average temperature of the season is 26.6°C.

(iii) Winter

November to February is the coldest season of the district. The average temperature of the season in the day is 27.8°C and in nights it may to 11.1°C.

Economic Profile

The economic system of the district is rural. The main avenue of the economy is agricultural products, bidi industries and some small-scale industries. This district is, still untouched by the economic development and modern civilisation of the country and the world even in the 21st century.

Tehsils, Blocks, Towns and Villages

The district at present comprises of 7 tehsils, 11 community development blocks, 11 towns and 2,086 villages.

Rivers

The Sagar district has four main rivers Bina, Dhasan, Bewas and Sonar.

Agriculture and Forest

Agriculture is the chief business of the district, which depends on the rain of monsoon. Main crops grown in the district are wheat, soyabean and chana. Khurai block of

Sagar district by the agricultural viewpoint is called as *"Punjab"* of Sagar. Soyabean is an economic crop of Sagar.

The district has total forest region of about 2999 sq. km, out of which 1916 sq. km is reserved forest 834.0 sq km is protected forest and 249.0 sq. km is unclassified forest.

Industrial Development

There are extreme lack of major industries in the district but Sagar has many cottage and small scale industries, i.e., the bidi making industries, agarbatti factories, soap factories, broom making and basket making factories, carpentry, blacksmithy, pottery, brass, steel utensils making, tiles and brick making, silver and gold ornaments making are very common in this town. Dal mills, and timber industries are very famous in this district.

Diversity of Population

The diversity in the morphological features of the population of this area is quite variable. Here the people are both fair to dark skin, medium short to tall stature and thin to thick lips are found. The texture of the hair varies from straight to wavy and often curly. This diversity shows that various ethnic strain have contributed to the present, diversified physical forms of this region's population.

Raj Gond

Among the 51 million of the tribal population of India as per 1981 census, there is no group more numerous and of greater historical importance than the people generally know by the genetic term 'Gond'. After them large region of the Decan is described as Gondwana, a name adopt also by geologist in the classification of middle Mesozoic and upper Paleozoic formations. The majority of Gonds are found, now a days in the state of Madhya Pradesh. Their main strong holds are the Satpura plateau including the district of Betul, Chhindwạra and Seoni where the western type of Gondi is spoken the district of Mandla, Jabalpur where the Gonds have adopted the local dialect of Hindi .

Until 1947, Gond rajas ruled on the state of Kawardha Sakti, Raigarh and Sarangarh, then Known as the *Chhhattisgarh state.*

The Raj Gond is tribal sub-division of Gond and originally a principal tribe of the Dravidian family. According to Gonds forsyth in many cases the Raj Gonds are the descendents of alliances between rajput adventures and Gonds. But the term Raj Gond practically comprises the landholding subdivision of the Gonds. The Raj Gonds rank with the Hindu cultivating castes and Brahmans take water from them. The three types of Gonds are found in Sagar district namely Raj Gonds, Khatulhas and Bhois, among them Raj Gonds are the superior land ruler and are found in large number.

They are claim to come in Sagar from Gujrat before Akbar's time. The Khatulha Gonds belonged to the old Gond principality of Khotola in Bijawa. They occasionally intermarry with Raj Gonds, though the later considers them as somewhat lower than themselves. The Bhoi Gonds are the most primitive members of the tribe. Gond, however, have a pride of their own and no outsider not even Bramhin or Rajput can become a Gond.

The Raj Gonds had adopted Hindu diets and rituals. They employ Kanaujiya and Sarwariya Brahmins for their ceremonies, wear the sacred thread and forbid widow marriage.

The Raj Gonds worship Sal Mohua, Mango and Achar trees and will not cut or burn them. Their principled God is Bura Deo, who is supposed to be live in Koha tree (Terminalia, Arjuna) in the forest.

Most of the tribal people abandoned their own language were as they also speaks a Bundelkhandi Hindi. The cloths are very simple, the ladies wear "Dhoti and Polka " and the Gents wear " Dhoti and Bandi ". They also wear Dhoti Kurta or Kamij when they go out side the village. The ornaments are made up of silver and gold. Every lady must have wear some ornaments according to her economic condition.

They are patrilineal and endogamous in nature. Nuclear and joint familes are also found.

The marriage ceremony is not complicated now days it is similar to the Hindu marriage system. As compared to the Hindu marriage the most distinctive feature of Gond marriage is that the procession usually, though not always starts from house of the bride and the main ceremony is preformed at the house of the bride groom. Infant marriage is not practised and the girl is as a matter of fact allowed a great deal more latitude in the choice of the husband.

The Gonds are the hardworking people though education ratio is low in them. The impact of modern ideas is increasing rapidly. They are very alert for their claims. They send their children to schools.

Most of the Raj Gonds have their own land. To supplement their income they resort to occasional agricultural and bidi labour. The source of additional income may come from selling vegetables, Tendu leaves, Sal seed etc. Which can be done by any member of the household although women predominantly conduct such business.

The staple food of the Raj Gonds comprises rice, millets and wild fruit. Vegetables include brinjals, potatoes, peas, beans, lady's finger, chillies, cabbage, cauliflower, radish, beet root, carrot and all the leafy vegetables. Non-vegetarian foods such as fish, goat meat and chicken are also taken as and when available. Liquor forms one of the most important constituents of their life. The frequency of liquor consumption depends upon the socio-economic status.

3
Material and Methodology

Universe of Study

Present study has been conducted among the Raj Gonds of Sagar district, Madhya Pradesh. The concern data as been collected from Raj Gonds predominated villages of Kesli, Rehli and Sagar blocks of Sagar district in which more than 70% of Raj Gonds population resides.

Sample Size

It has been estimated by population progression method based on 1981 census that near about 10359 eligible couples including blood related couples (aged between 15 - 49 years) residing in this district.

For investigation 300 unrelated couples (which cover near about 2.8% of the population) were randomly selected for the fruitful results.

Sampling Frame

The village of these blocks having Raj Gonds has been arranged in descending order on the basis of their population. The village having greater concentration was selected by probability proportion. From these villages different sample has been taken but the sample size of each village under study varies on the basis of their population in order to make the sample a representative one. Data were collected from twenty five villages namely Apchand, Barpani, Dhura, Padariya, Bada Piperiya in Sagar block,

Kadta, Jamuniya Sahajpuri Kalan, Semra Gond, Tada Datpura, Murga, Parasiya in Rehli Block and Chauka, Ghana, Tumri, Jamunia, Ramgarha, Jamuniya near Charka, Kachhaua, Anghori Duhli, Nandiya in Kesli Block. A unrelated nuclear family formed the basic unit of study and every alternate household was undertaken for the their investigation. The husband and wife were taken as the main subjects for this study. In case of non-availability or non-cooperation the next unrelated family was taken up for the study. In all, as per the sampling design we were able to collect data on socio-cultural practices, socio-biological practices and genetical parameters of 300 families following the above mentioned rigid sample design. While collecting the data following criteria are followed (1) All the related families were excluded from the study sample. (2) Single parent families were excluded. (3) Families where the mothers were found infertile were eliminated from the study sample. (4) Families, where accidental deaths of the children occurred within one year of their birth were excluded.

Tools of Data Collection

On the basis of the preliminary field survey and observation, semi structured schedule was prepared and pretested to estimate the feasibility component during data collection. Besides obtaining information on identity location etc. the schedule was designed to get in depth information of about the village level organization, family level organisation among the Raj Gonds.

Determination of Age

Generally in rural areas estimation of age of people is often very difficult. Therefore for age determination of the subject, recall method of social event, in concern area.

Data Collection

The information regarding reproductive and child

health care practices was collected with the help of structured schedule, observation and case study method. The in-depth information on reproductive and child health care performance was collected by drawing extended genealogies with pregnancy to pregnancy enumeration recording out come of each pregnancy. The provided information by the couple was cross checked by interviewing the elderly people of the village. Attempts were made to cross check information on the reproductive wastage from local dais, trained birth attendants and other health functionaries to strengthen the validity of data.

Statistical Method Used

Gene frequencies were calculated by using the formula given by Mourant (1976). The data were arranged using the FOXPLUS data base package and the simple chi square contingency tables were used for finding out significance by the microstate and SPSS statistical package.

4
Findings

Reproductive and Child Health Profile

Table 4.1 reveals literacy level among the Raj Gonds in which 80.67% women and 56.33% men cannot read and write whereas 19.33% women and 43.66% men can.

Table 4.1 : Details of Literacy Level

Total families	Wife				Husband			
	Writing		Reading		Writing		Reading	
	Yes	No	Yes	No	Yes	No	Yes	No
300	58	242	58	242	131	169	131	169
%	19.33%	80.67%	19.33%	80.67%	43.67%	56.33%	43.67%	53.33%

Table 4.2 shows that per mother number of children among Raj Gonds in which most of the women have two children (29.33%) followed by one (28.00%), five (10.67%), three (10.00%), four (9.33%), six (7.67%), seven (3.00%) and eight 2.00 per cent.

Table 4.2 : Details of Per Mother Number of Children

Number of women	Number of children								No Children
	One	Two	Three	Four	Five	Six	Seven	Eight	
300	84	88	30	28	32	23	9	6	-
%	28.00%	29.33%	10.00%	9.33%	10.67%	7.67%	3.00%	2.00%	-

The mortality profile of the Raj Gond mothers is shown in Table 4.3. It is revealed from the table that out of total pregnancies, live births are most frequent (93.82%) followed by abortions (6.17%), still births (12.73%), child death (9.00%) and juvenile death (5.64%), infant death rate is found highest (13.55) than child death rate (9.59), adolescent death rate (6.01) and reproductive wastage 6.17.

Table 4.4 shows the abortion profile of the Raj Gond mothers. It could be observed from the table that 16.33% women respondents have faced abortions in which all the cent percent abortions were self abortions. Out of them 49.25% women were aborted once followed by 20.89% twice and 2.98% thrice.

Table 4.5 reveals that out of the women who faced abortions, 38.76% suffered from excess bleeding with in one week after abortion followed by 10.20% from high fever and 2.04% from fouls smelling while 48.98% have all problems.

Table 4.6 shows the details place of treatment for the problems faced after abortion by Raj Gond mothers. It could be observed from the table that, out of them 77.55% didn't take any consultation or treatment after abortion while 4.08% women have consulted with health worker or primary health centre or elder ladies, rest of the 10.20% women went to private doctor for their problems.

Table 4.7 shows the birth order wise still births profile among the Raj Gond mothers. It could be observed from the table that, women who faced still births are 3.67%, out of which 21.43% cases were found in fifth pregnancy followed by 14.28% in second, fourth, seventh & eighth rest of 7.14% case were found in third & sixth pregnancy.

Table 4.3 : Details of Mortality Profile

Number of women	*Number of women become pregnant in their life time*	*Number of total pregnancies*	*Number of abortion & still births*	*Number of live births*	*Number of child deaths (1day - 1 years)*	*Number of children death*	*Number of juvenile death*	*Infant death rate*	*Children death rate*	*Adolescent death rate*	*Reproductive wastage rate*
300	300	1311	81	1230	167	118	74	-	-	-	-
% / Rate			6.18%	93.82%	12.74%	9.00%	5.64%	13.58	9.59	6.01	6.18

Table 4.4 : Details of Abortion Profile

Number of women	Women having abortions	Type of abortion			Number of abortions			
		Induced	Self	Total	One	Two	Three	No response
300	49	-	67	67	33	14	2	-
%	16.33%	-	100.00%	100.00%	49.25%	20.89%	2.88%	-

Table 4.5 : Health Problems Faced within one Week after Abortion

Number of women	Number of women having self abortions	Excess bleeding	High fever	Foul smelling	Bleed-ing	Weak-ness	Head-ache	Back pain	Abdo-men pain	All problems
300	49	19	5	1	-	-	-	-	-	24
%	16.33%	38.76%	10.20%	2.04%	-	-	-	-	-	48.98%

Table 4.6 : Place of Treatment for the Problems Faced after Abortion

Number of women	Number of women having self abortions	Yes									No treatment
		Government hospital	Primary health center (PHC)	Private doctor	Health worker	Government nurse	Auxiliary nurse midwife (ANM)	Elderly ladies	Dai	Others	
300	49	-	2	5	2	-	-	2	-	-	38
%	16.33%	-	4.08%	10.20%	4.08%	-	-	4.08%	-	-	77.55%

Table 4.7 : Birth Order-wise Still Births

Number of women	Still birth			Birth order wise still birth situation							
	Yes	No	No reply	One	Two	Three	Four	Five	Six	Seven	Eighth
300	11	289	-	-	2	1	2	3	1	2	2
%	3.67%	96.33%	-	-	14.28%	7.14%	14.28%	21.43%	7.14%	14.28%	14.28%

Table 4.8 reveals that in last seven years (1996 - 2002) 95.33% women become pregnant. Total 343 pregnancies were known in this period. 19.00% women become twice in these years. Highest frequency of pregnancies 19.53% is found in year 2000 followed by 17.20% in year 2001, 16.32% in year 1999 while lowest frequency is observed 6.70% in year 2002.

Table 4.9 reveals that 34.00% women respondents were visited by Auxiliary nurse midwife (A.N.M.) during pregnancy while 66.00% were not visited.

Table 4.10 reveals that out of 34.00% women visited of Auxiliary Nurse Midwife (ANM) maximum 25.49% women were visited in seventh month followed by 22.55% in eight and fourth month respectively and six month (13.72%), while only 2.94% were visited in third month of pregnancy.

Table 4.11 reveals that 4.67% women respondent were advised for health checkup by Auxiliary Nurse Midwife (ANM) while 89.33% were not advised and rest of 6.00% have forgotten about it.

Table 4.12 reveals that during pregnancy no women use sex identification techniques for identify sex of a baby in her womb.

Table 4.13 reveals that during pregnancy only 12.00% took their body weight, only 7.33% went for blood pressure checkup and only 34.00% have taken iron and folic acid tablets.

Table 4.14 reveals that out of 34.00% women who took iron and folic acid tablets 50.98% women were advised & given two tablets for a day followed by 37.25% one tablet and 3.92% three tablet whereas 7.84% women did not remember the number of tablets per day.

Table 4.15 reveals that 14.33% women have received

Table 4.8 : Year-wise Pregnancies (last seven years)

Number of women	*No pregnancy*	*Number of pregnant women respondent*							*Total number of preg-nancies*	*Two time preg-nant in this period*	*No reply*
		1996	*1997*	*1998*	*1999*	*2000*	*2001*	*2002*	*1996 - 2002*		
300	14	38	52	48	56	67	59	23	343	57	-
%	4.67%	11.08%	15.16%	13.99%	16.33%	19.53%	17.20%	6.70%	100.00%	19.00%	-

Table 4.9 : Visit of Auxiliary Nurse Midwife (ANM) during Pregnancy

Number of women respondent	*Visited by auxiliary nurse midwife (ANM)*	
	Yes	*No*
300 %	102 34.00%	198 66.00%

Table 4.10 : Month wise Visits of Auxiliary Nurse Midwife (ANM) during Pregnancy

Number of women	*Number of women visited by auxiliary nurse midwife (ANM) during pregnancy*	*Month of pregnancy*								
		First	*Second*	*Third*	*Fourth*	*Fifth*	*Sixth*	*Seventh*	*Eighth*	*Ninth*
300	102	4	6	3	14	12	14	26	23	-
%	34.00%	3.92%	5.88%	2.94%	13.73%	11.76%	13.73%	25.49%	22.55%	-

tetanus toxied injection during pregnancy where as 85.66% have not received.

Table 4.11 : Women Advised for Health Checkup by Auxiliary Nurse Midwife (ANM)

Number of women	*Health check up advised*		
	Yes	*No*	*Not remember*
300	14	268	18
%	4.67%	89.33%	6.00%

Table 4.12 : Utilization of Sex Determination Technique before Delivery

Number of women	*Use of sex identification technique*		
	Yes	*No*	*No reply*
300	0	300	0
%	-	100.00%	-

Table 4.13 : During Pregnancy Availed Health Care Facilities

Number of women	Body weight		Blood pressure		Iron & folic acid tablets		
	Yes	No	Yes	No	Yes	No	No reply
300	36	264	22	278	102	192	6
%	12.00%	88.00%	7.33%	92.67%	34.00%	64.00%	2.00%

Table 4.14 : Details of Number of Iron & Folic Acid Tablets given to Pregnant Women to Eat Per Day during Pregnancy

Number of women	Number of women given iron & folic acid tablets	Number of tablets advised and given for a day						Not Remember
		One	Two	Three	Four	Five	Six	
300	102	38	52	4	-	-	-	8
%	34.00%	37.25%	50.98%	3.92%	-	-	-	7.84%

Table 4.15 : Details of Availed Tetanus Toxied Immunization During Pregnancy

Number of women	Tetanus toxid immunisation	
	Yes	No
300	43	257
%	14.33%	85.67%

Table 4.16 reveals that out of these 14.33% women, 90.69 % have given one tetanus toxied injection while 9.30% have received two.

Table 4.17 reveals that during pregnancy Raj Gond mothers have faced various health problems. Swollen in hand and feet is found most frequent (35.33%) followed by weakness (14.00%), tiredness (11.33%), heaviness (7.66%) not feeling well (6.667%), eye problem (1.33%), bleeding (1.00%) and no sensation of embryo movement

Table 4.16 : Details of Number of Tetanus Toxied Injection received by Women during Pregnancy

Total mother	Number of women received tetanus injection	Number of tetanus toxied injections received				
		One	Two	Three	Four	Not remember
300	43	39	4	-	-	-
%	14.33%	90.70%	9.30%	-	-	-

(0.33%), whereas 5.33% women faced other problems, 15.33% faced more than one problem and 2.66% did not reply the question.

Table 4.18 reveals that during pregnancy 17.67% women have utilized health care services whereas 71.00% did not utilize and 11.33% women did not face any problem.

Table 4.19 reveals that out of 17.67% women who took treatment for problems during pregnancy, 50.94% have visited to private doctor followed by 28.30% health workers and 20.75% government doctors.

Table 4.20 reveals that during pregnancy only 1.33% women were advised for regular health checkup by health workers. The 75.33% respondent have paid government fee for health checkup while 24.67% have got free checkup

Table 4.21 reveals that most of the deliveries i.e., 94.33% were conducted at home with the help of elder ladies followed by 4.00% at primary health center and 1.66% at District hospital.

Table 4.22 reveals that delivery instruments were not available in 94.33% cases while in 5.67% cases instruments were available.

Table 4.23 reveals that during delivery only 26.33% women have suffered with various health problems. Pain before delivery is most frequent problem reported by 60.76% followed by pains with short intervals of time by 15.19%,

Table 4.17 : Types of Health Problem faced during Pregnancy

Number of women	*Swollen in hands & feet*	*Weak-ness*	*Tired-ness*	*Heavi-ness*	*Eye problem*	*Bleed-ing*	*No sensation of embryo movement*	*Not feeling well*	*Others*	*More than one problem*	*No reply*
300	106	42	34	23	4	3	1	17	16	46	8
%	35.33%	14.00%	11.33%	7.67%	1.33%	1.00%	0.33%	5.67%	5.33%	15.33%	2.67%

not feeling well by 11.39% and pains of longer duration by 8.86% women.

Table 4.18 : Utilization of Health Care Services during Pregnancy

Number of women	Treatment received		No problem
	Yes	No	
300	53	213	34
%	17.67%	71.00%	11.33%

Table 4.19 : Utilized Place for the Treatment of Health Problems during Pregnancy

Number of women	Number of women received treatment	Government doctor	Private doctor	Health worker	Nurse	Dai	No reply
300	53	11	27	15	-	-	-
%	17.67%	20.75%	50.94%	28.30%	-	-	-

Table 4.20 : Services given by Health Worker during Pregnancy

Number of women	Advise of regular health cheek up by health worker			Health checkup payment	
	Yes	No	No reply	No fee	Only government fee
300	4	296	-	74	226
%	1.33%	98.67%	-	24.67%	75.33%

Table 4.21 : Details of Place of Delivery.

Number of women	Primary health center (PHC)	District hospital	Private hospital	Home			
				By			Total
				Doctor	Nurse	Elder ladies	
300	12	5	-	-	-	283	283
%	4.00%	1.67%	-	-	-	94.33%	94.33%

Table 4.24 reveals that in 82.67% deliveries new blade has been used as a tool for cutting navel cord followed by old blades in 8.00% & knife in 3.67% cases while in 5.67%

Table 4.23 : Details of Type of Health Problems faced by Women during Delivery.

Number of women	No	Yes	Health Problems					No reply
			Pain before	Pains with short interval	Pain of longer duration	Not feeling	Others	
300	221	79	48	12	7	9	3	-
%	73.67%	26.33%	60.76%	15.19%	8.86%	11.39%	3.78%	-

cases other instruments have been used. Out of these in only 12.67% cases the tool has been boiled before using where as in 82.00% it has been used without boiled and 5.33% women didn't reply this question.

Table 4.24 : Details of Instruments used for Cutting Navel Cord

Number of women	Used instrument				Used instruments boiled in water		
	Blade new	Blade old	Knife	Others	Yes	No	No reply
300	248	24	11	17	38	246	16
%	82.67%	8.00%	3.67%	5.67%	12.67%	82.00%	5.33%

Table 4.25 reveals that after one week of delivery 75.67% women have suffered with various health problems. Out of these health problem back pain in 23.79% respondents is most frequent followed by headache 17.18%, high fever 16.74% while foul smelling is least frequent in 1.32% women.

Table 4.26 reveals that out of 75.67% women who have faced health problems after delivery only 23.55% have utilize treatment facilities while 76.65% did not take treatment 50.94% treated women consulted private doctors followed by 28.80% Auxiliary Nurse Midwife (A.N.M) and 20.75% and government doctor.

Table 4.25 : Details of Health Problems Faced after one Week of Delivery

Number of women	*No*	*Yes*	*Health Problems*								
			Excess bleeding	*High fever*	*Heaviness*	*Foul smelling*	*Cerveous secretion*	*Weakness*	*Headache*	*Back pain*	*Others*
300	73	227	12	38	26	3	9	22	39	54	24
%	24.33%	75.67%	5.29%	16.74%	11.45%	1.32%	3.96%	9.69%	17.18%	23.79%	10.57%

Table 4.26 : Details of Utilization of Available Health Care Services

Number of women	*Number of women faced health problems*	*Is utilized treatment facilities*			*Treatment Place*					
		No	*Yes*	*No reply*	*Government doctors*	*Private doctors*	*Auxiliary nurse midwife (ANM)*	*Magico-religious treatment*	*Dai*	*Others*
300	227	174	53	-	11	27	15	-	-	-
%	75.67%	76.65%	23.35%	-	20.75%	50.94%	28.30%	-	-	-

Table 4.27 reveals that seventy two per cent women were not visited by any health worker after delivery followed by 28.00% women respondent reported visit of health workers. Out of them 45.24% reported one visit followed by 17.86% two visit than 15.48% three visit, 14.29% four visit, 7.14 five visit and distributed medicines to 92.86% women's.

Table 4.27 : Details of Visit of Health Workers after Delivery

Number of women	*Visited*		*Number of visit*					*Distributed medicines*	
	No	*Yes*	*One*	*Two*	*Three*	*Four*	*Five*	*Yes*	*No*
300	216	84	38	15	13	12	6	78	6
%	72.00%	28.00%	45.24	17.86%	15.48%	14.29%	7.14%	92.86%	7.143%

Table 4.28 reveals that only 32.67% women have various reproductive health problems. Out of them burning sensation in urinal is most frequent problem by 47.96% women and 12.24% suffering with vaginal secretion. Secretion type is thin white or thick brown white in 16.67% cases while thick white in 8.33% cases. In women suffering with vaginal secretion 23.47% have back pain and 15.30% have fever due to secretion. Other health problems with buring sensation in vagina are found in 9.18% case and pain during intercourse in 8.16% cases.

Table 4.29 reveals that out of 32.62% women having reproductive health problems, 32.65% have conversation with their husband followed by 23.47% women with mother or mother in law, 9.18% with elderly ladies. A large number of women i.e., 24.98% don't share their problem with any one due of hesitation.

Table 4.30 reveals that out of 32.62% women who reproductive health problems, 28.57% have consultation with private doctor 28.57% followed by 23.46% with Auxiliary Nurse Midwife (ANM) while 18.37% do not take

Table 4.28 : Details of Reproductive Health Problems in Women

Number of women	*Number of women faced health problems*	*Health problems*					
		Burning sensation in urinal		*Pain during intercourse*		*Vaginal secretion*	
		Yes	*No*	*Yes*	*No*	*Yes*	*No*
1	2	3	4	5	6	7	8
300	98	47	51	8	90	12	86
%	32.67%	47.96%	52.04%	8.16%	91.84%	12.24%	87.76%

...Continued

Type of vaginal secretion				*Burning / wounds in vagina*			*Problems due to secretion*			
							Back pain		*Fever*	
9	10	11	12	13	14	15	16	17	18	19
Thick smelled liquid in small quantity secretion	*Thick white secretion*	*Thin white secretion*	*Thick brown white secretion*	*Burn-ing*	*Wou-nds*	*Noth-ing*	*Yes*	*No*	*Yes*	*No*
7	1	2	2	9	-	89	23	75	15	83
58.33%	8.33%	16.67%	16.67%	9.18%	-	90.82%	23.47%	76.53%	15.30%	84.69%

any treatment for problems and 3.06% utilise traditional treatment.

Table 4.29 : Details of Conversation with Whom Regarding Health Problems by Women

Number of women	*Number of women faced health problems*	*Mother or Mother in law*	*Dai*	*Nurse*	*Elder ladies*	*Husband*	*Others*	*Don't tell any because of hesitation*
300	98	23	4	-	9	32	7	24
%	32.62%	23.47%	4.08%	-	9.18%	32.65%	7.14%	24.49%

Table 4.31 reveals that out of total respondent 37.67% women have knowledge about Acquired Immune Deficiency Syndrome (AIDS) and 5.33% women did not reply. Out of these aware women 37.17% get this knowledge through radio followed by 30.09% by husband, 14.15% by friends, 11.50% by television & 3.54% by dais.

Table 4.32 reveals that out of these 37.67% women those are aware to AIDS, 25.66% think that heterosexuality is the mode of transmission of AIDS. According to 21.24% women intercourse and 5.30% kissing can transmitted AIDS while 10.62% women knows that unhygienic activities can transmit it followed by 15.92% sleeping with infected person and 7.96% by the use of others used needle.

Table 4.33 reveals that out of the women who are aware of AIDS 27.43% know that AIDS can be prevent, but 42.48% do not know about medium of its prevention while condom is the preventive medium for 23.53% women followed by safe intercourse for 8.82% women and blood test before donation for 5.88% women whereas 61.76% answered all these medium.

Table 4.34 reveals that 29.33% women are aware to sexually transmitted diseases while 5.34% women didn't

Table 4.30 : Place of Health Services for the Treatment of Health roblems

Number of women	Number of women faced health problems	Place of treatment										
		Government doctor	Private doctor	Auxi-liary nurse mid-wife	Medi-cal shop	Dai	Tradi-tional treat-ment	Friend or Relative	Self treat-ment	Oth-ers	No treat-ment	No reply
300	98	11	28	23	2	-	3	-	-	-	18	13
%	32.67%	11.22%	28.57%	23.47%	2.04%	-	3.06%	-	-	-	18.37%	13.26%

Table 4.31 : Source of Awareness Regarding Acquired Immune Deficiency Disease Syndrome (AIDS)

Number of women	*Awareness of AIDS*			*Source of awareness*			
	No	*Yes*	*No reply*	*Radio*	*Television*	*Newspaper*	*Magazines*
1	2	3	4	5	6	7	8
300	171	113	16	42	13	-	-
%	57.00%	37.67%	5.33%	37.17%	11.50%	-	-
...Continued							
Dai	*Nurse*	*Doctor*	*Relatives*	*Friends*	*Husbands*	*Posters*	*Others*
9	10	11	12	13	14	15	16
4	-	-	-	16	34	-	4
3.54%	-	-	-	14.16%	30.09%	-	3.54%

Table 4.32: Details of Awareness About the Mode of Transmission of Acquired Immuno Deficiency Syndrome (AIDS)

Number of women	*Number of women having awareness of acquired immune deficiency syndrome*	*Transmission medium*					
		Homo-sexuality	*Heterosexuality*			*By the use of others used needle*	*By the use of others used cloth or blade*
			Inter-course	*Kiss*	*Both*		
1	2	3	4	5	6	7	8
300	113	-	24	6	29	9	2
%	37.67%	-	21.24%	5.31%	25.66%	7.96%	1.77%

... Continued

By infected mother to her children	*By unhygienic activities*	*By infected persons blood transmission*	*By infected persons pushing*	*By Infected persons hand-shaking*	*By infected persons with eating*	*By infected persons with sleeping*
9	10	11	12	13	14	15
6	12	2	-	-	5	18
5.31%	10.62%	1.77%	-	-	4.42%	15.93%

Table 4.33 : Details of Awareness about the Prevention Acquired Immune Deficiency Syndrome (AIDS) from Transmission

Number of women	*Number of women aware of AIDS*	*Is prevention of AIDS possible*		*Medium of prevention*						
		No	*Yes*	*Condom*	*Safe intercourse*	*Checkup of blood before transmission*	*Use of boiled needle*	*By preventing AIDS suffering women from getting pregnant*	*By all*	*Not know*
300	113	31	34	8	3	2	-	-	21	48
%	37.67%	27.43%	30.09%	23.53%	8.82%	5.88%	-	-	61.76%	42.48%

Table 4.34 : Source of Awareness for Sexually Transmitted Diseases (STD)

Number of women	*Awareness of STD disease*			*Source of awareness*			
	No	*Yes*	*No reply*	*Radio*	*Television*	*Newspaper*	*Magazines*
1	2	3	4	5	6	7	8
300	196	88	16	17	4	-	-
%	65.33%	29.33%	5.34%	19.32%	4.55%	-	-

...Continued

Dai	*Health worker*	*Doctor*	*Relatives*	*Friends*	*Husbands*	*Posters*	*Others*
9	10	11	12	13	14	15	16
14	12	8	-	12	19	-	2
15.91%	13.64%	9.09%	-	13.64%	21.59%	-	2.27%

reply the question. Women those are aware, out of them 21.59% got information by their husbands followed by 19.31% from radio and 13.64% by health workers or friends.

Table 4.35 reveals that a large percentage of women i.e., 64.67% is aware about malaria. Out of them husband is the source of knowledge in 24.74% cases followed by radio in 23.71% cases and malaria workers in 16.49% cases.

Table 4.36 reveals that out of these respondents 16.00% women were pregnant at the time of data collection.

Table 4.37 reveals that 61.00% women thinks child-birth can be limited and 39.00% thinks that it is not possible. In 61.00% women, for 33.88% condom is the best medium to limit childbirth followed by 19.67% reported oral pills than 15.84% sterilization while 30.60% all these methods.

Table 4.38 reveals that at the time data collection 49.33% respondents were using family welfare device. Out of them in 42.57% cases husbands & in 26.35% cases wives were using devices while in 31.08% cases both husbands & wives were using family welfare device.

Table 4.39 reveals that out of these 49.33% respondents using family welfare device, 64.19% were using condom followed by 14.18% tubectomy, 12.16% oral pills, 8.10% safe period and 1.35% vasectomy method.

Table 4.40 reveals that Women who have information about family welfare devices are 61.00%. For 36.06% of them husband was the source of information followed by 26.23% radio, 15.30% A.N.M., 13.11% friends and 9.29% television.

Table 4.41 reveals that out of these 49.33% respondents using family welfare device 21.62% women were facing

Table 4.35 : Source of Awareness for Malaria

Number of women	*Awareness about malaria*			*Source of awareness*			
	No	*Yes*	*No reply*	*Radio*	*Television*	*Newspaper*	*Magazines*
1	2	3	4	5	6	7	8
300	106	194	-	46	17	-	-
%	35.33%	64.67%	-	23.71%	8.76%	-	-

...Continued

Dai	*Malaria worker*	*Doctor*	*Relatives*	*Friends*	*Husbands*	*Posters*	*Others*
9	10	11	12	13	14	15	16
6	32	24	-	21	48	-	-
3.09%	16.49%	12.37%	-	10.82%	24.74%	-	-

Table 4.36 : Status of Presently Pregnant Women

Number of women	Number of pregnant women	Number of non pregnant women
300	48	252
%	16.00%	84.00%

Table 4.37 : Awareness about Family Welfare Devices

Number of women	Can child birth limited		Medium of limiting child birth						
	Yes	No	Oral pills	Copper-T	Condom	Loop	Injection	Sterilization	All
300	183	117	36	-	62	-	-	29	56
%	61.00%	39.00%	19.67%	-	33.88%	-	-	15.85%	30.60%

Table 4.38 : Details of Utilisation of Family Welfare Devices (presently by whom)

Number of women	Utilized		By husband	By wife	By both
	No	Yes			
300	152	148	63	39	46
%	50.67%	49.33%	42.57%	26.35%	31.08%

Table 4.39 : Details of Presently Utilized Family Welfare Devices

Number of families	Number of families presently utilising family welfare devices	Oral pills	Copper-T	Condom	Vasectomy	Tubectomy	Intra uterine devices	Safe period	Others
300	148	18	-	95	2	21	-	12	-
%	49.33%	12.16%	-	64.19%	1.35%	14.19%	-	8.11%	-

Table 4.40 : Source of Awareness for Family Welfare Devices

Number of women	*Number of women aware of family welfare devices*	*Source of awareness*					
		Television	*Radio*	*Newspaper*	*Magazines*	*Posters*	*Auxiliary Nurse Midwife (ANM)*
1	2	3	4	5	6	7	8
300	183	17	48	-	-	-	28
%	61.00%	9.29%	26.23%	-	-	-	15.30%

...Continued

Doctor	*Dai*	*Relatives*	*Friends*	*Husbands*	*Health worker*	*Others*
9	10	11	12	13	14	15
-	-	-	24	66	-	-
-	-	-	13.11%	36.06%	-	-

Table 4.41 : Details of Advice of Health Worker for Problem Arises during the use of Family Welfare Devices

Total number of women	*Number of women utilizing of family welfare devices*	*Health problem faced*		*Type of health problems*			
		Yes	*No*	*Body/ back pain*	*Fatness*	*Heaviness*	*Sensation of vomiting*
1	2	3	4	5	6	7	8
300	148	32	116	19	4	2	6
%	49.33%	21.62%	78.38%	59.37%	12.50%	6.25%	18.76%

...Continued

Angriness in inhaling	*Irregular menstrual cycle*	*Excess bleeding*	*White secretion*	*Clot secretion*	*Unsatisfiction*	*Others*
9	10	11	12	13	14	15
-	1	-	-	-	-	-
-	3.12%	-	-	-	-	-

Table 4.42 : Details of Place of Treatment for Problems Arises during the use of Family Welfare Devices

Number of women	*Number of women having health problem*	*Get treatment*		*Place of treatment*					
		No	*Yes*	*Government doctor*	*Private doctor*	*Auxiliary nurse midwife*	*Dai*	*Friend / Relative*	*Self treatment*
300	32	21	11	2	9	-	-	-	-
%	10.67%	65.63%	34.38%	18.18%	81.82%	-	-	-	-

health problems due to use of family welfare device. Body or back pain is most frequent reported by 59.37% women followed by 18.76% reported vomiting sensation than 12.50% fattiness, 6.25% heaviness and 3.12% irregular menstrual cycle.

Table 4.42 reveals that women who have health problems due to use of family welfare device were 21.62% of presently users. Out of them 34.38% have taken treatment in which 81.82% women get treatment from private doctor while 18.18% from government doctor.

Table 4.43 reveals that out of these 49.33% women 58.11% were not satisfied with the family welfare devices they were using while 41.89% were satisfied.

Table 4.43 : Opinion of Women Regarding the Satisfactory Utilisation of Family Welfare Devices.

Number women	Number of women utilised of family welfare devices	Yes	No
300	148	62	86
%	49.33%	41.89%	58.11%

Table 4.44 reveals that place chosen for tubectomy was camp by 10.14% women while 4.05% women were sterilization in primary health center.

Table 4.44 : Details of place of tubectomy

Number of women	Number of women utilised of family welfare devices	Utilised tubectomy		Place of tubectomy		
		Not used	Used	Primary health center PHC)	Camp	District hospital
300	148	127	21	6	15	-
%	49.33%	85.81%	14.19%	4.05%	10.14%	-

Table 4.45 reveals that at the time of data collection 49.33% women were using family welfare devices. For 69.59% of them devices are easily available from female health worker and for 3.38% these are not available easily on shop while 16.22% women did not answer the question.

Table 4.45 : Details of Availability of Family Welfare Devices

Number of women	*Number of women utilizing of family welfare devices*	*Easily available*	*Not regularly available in primary health center (PHC)*	*Not easily available from female health worker*	*Not easily available on shop*	*No reply*
300	148	103	-	16	5	24
%	49.33%	69.59%	-	10.81%	3.38%	16.22%

Table 4.46 reveals that out of these 50.67% respondent who were not using family welfare devices at the time of data collection only 34.87% have used them in past. In 43.40% cases device was used by husband while in 33.96% cases it was used by wives. 43.40% couples used condoms followed by 33.96% used oral pills and 22.64% used safe period.

Table 4.47 reveals that in these women 35.53% were presently not using due to unsatisfaction followed by 27.63% unsatisfaction by devices, 11.84% expecting children and 8.55% due to body or back pain, while 1.97% were not utilising device due to difficulty in use and 1.32% due to irregular menstrual cycle.

Table 4.48 reveals that out of these 50.67% respondent not using any family welfare devices at the time of data collection and only 24.34% respondent devices were distributed by health worker while 75.66% did not get these devices.

Table 4.46 : Detaiis of utilization of the family welfare devices in past who are presently nonuscr.

Number women	Number of women presently nonuser of family welfare devices	Utilized in past		By			Types				Intra uterine devices	Safe period	Others
		No	Yes	Wife	Husband	Both	Oral pills	Co-per-T	Con-dom	Loop			
300	152	99	53	18	23	12	18	-	23	-	-	12	-
%	50.67%	65.13%	34.87%	33.96%	43.40%	22.64%	33.96%	-	43.40%	-	-	22.64%	-

Table 4.47 : Details about Reason for Presently not Utilising Family Welfare Devices

Number of women	*Number of women not utilising family welfare devices*	*Reasons*						
		Willingness for children	*Unsatisfaction*	*Unavailability*	*Available by difficulty*	*Body or back pain*	*Fatness*	*Heaviness*
1	2	3	4	5	6	7	8	9
300	152	18	42	-	-	13	4	9
%	50.67%	11.84%	27.63%	-	-	8.55%	2.63%	5.92%

...Continued

Vomiting sensation	*Angriness in inhaling*	*Irregular menstrual cycle*	*Excess bleeding*	*White secretion*	*Clot secretion*	*Unsatisfiction*	*Difficulty in use*
10	11	12	13	14	15	16	17
7	-	2	-	-	-	54	3
4.61%	-	1.32%	-	-	-	35.53%	1.97%

Table 4.48 : Distribution of Family Welfare Devices by Health Worker

Number of women	Number of women not presently utilising any family welfare devices	Distributed	
		Yes	No
300	152	37	115
%	50.67%	24.34%	75.66%

Table 4.49 reveals that 61.00% of respondent mentioned that family welfare device are easily available while 17.67% didn't have any information about its availability while 21.33% mention devices are not available.

Table 4.49 : Availability of family welfare devices

Number of women respondent	Available		
	Yes	No	Not known
300	·183	64	53
%	61.00%	21.33%	17.67%

Table 4.50 reveals that 57.33% respondent were interested in utilising family welfare device. In which, 45.35% respondent were choose condom followed by 31.40% tubectomy, 12.21% safe period, 9.88% oral pills and 1.16% vasectomy.

Table 4.51 reveals that out of 50.67% women not using any family welfare devices. 23.03% were not using it because they don't like to use it followed by 15.13% due to unawareness, 9.21% thinks it is antireligious 8.55% feared about power loss, 3.95% because of husband's opposition & 1.32% due to family opposition.

Table 4.52 reveals that in 42.00% respondents family, head of the family is the decision maker for sterilization followed by their husband in 32.97% families, herself in 8.00% families, and in 2.00% families mother-in-law while 13.67% women did not answer the question.

Table 4.50 : Details of Preference for type of Family Welfare Devices in Utilisation

Number of women	Interested to utilise		Oral pills	Copper-T	Condom	Loop	Intra uterine devices	Safe period	Vasectomy	Tubectomy
	No	Yes								
300	128	172	17	-	78	-	-	21	2	54
%	42.67%	57.33%	9.88%	-	45.35%	-	-	12.21%	1.16%	31.40%

Table 4.51 : Detail of Socio-economic Reasons for Presently not Utilizing Family Welfare Devices

Number of women	*Number of women not utilising family welfare devices*	*Reasons*						
		Unawareness	*Antireli-gious*	*Family opposition*	*Husbands opposition*	*Elderly ladies*	*Unliking for use*	*Fear of sterilisation*
1	2	3	4	5	6	7	8	9
300	152	23	14	2	6	8	35	8
%	50.67%	15.13%	9.21%	1.32%	3.95%	5.26%	23.03%	5.26%

...Continued

Fear of power loss	*Fear of side effects of sterilization*	*Not available free*	*More costly*	*Difficulty in availability*	*Fear of their side effect in getting pregnant*	*All reasons*	*No reply*
10	11	12	13	14	15	16	17
13	4	-	-	-	-	39	-
8.55%	2.63%	-	-	-	-	25.66%	-

Table 4.52 : Detail of decision making persons for sterilization

Number of women	*Decision maker*						
	Husband	*Self*	*Mother in law*	*Sister in law*	*Head of the family*	*Other*	*No reply*
300	98	24	2	-	126	9	41
%	32.67%	8.00%	0.67%	-	42.00%	3.00%	13.67%

Table 4.53 reveals that 41.33% respondents were agreed for tubectomy while 58.67% were not.

Table 4.53 : Details of Opinion of Female for Tubectomy

Number of women respondent	*Agreed for tubectomy*	
	Yes	*No*
300	124	176
%	41.33%	58.67%

Table 4.54 reveals that health worker have visited 44.67% respondents in last three months while 48.33% were not visited and 7.00% did not remember. In 58.21% cases visits were taken by aganwadi worker rest of 41.79% by doctor. Out of 44.67% women who were visited by health worker 64.93% were satisfied with their visits.

Table 4.55 reveals that primary health centre was utilising by 24.67% women and only 37.84% were satisfied with the treatment facilities of centre while 62.16% were unsatisfied.

Table 4.56 reveals that primary health center is easily reachable for 35.33% women while not approachable for 64.67% women. According to 49.33% women medical

Table 4.54 : Health Worker Visit in Last Three Months

Number of women	*Visits of health worker*			*Visits are taken by*				
	Yes	*No*	*Not remember*	*Auxiliary nurse midwife (ANM)*	*Doctor*	*Aganwadi worker*	*Dai*	*Other*
1	2	3	4	5	6	7	8	9
300	134	145	21	-	56	78	-	-
%	44.67%	48.33%	7.00%	-	41.79%	58.21%	-	-

...Continued

Are you satisfied by the time given by these health worker	
No	*Yes*
10	11
47	87
35.07%	64.93%

Table 4.55 : Details of Utilization of Primary Health Center (PHC)

Utilisation of primary health centre (PHC)		*Treatment status*	
Yes	*No*	*Satisfied*	*Unsatisfied*
74	226	28	46
24.67%	75.33%	37.84%	62.16%

facilities are available in primary health centre. 78.00% women thinks that they have to wait for a long time in PHC. According to 41.33% women medicines are distributed in PHC. Behaviour of health workers and doctors of primary health centre was satisfactory for 42.67% women while it is unsatisfactory for 31.00% women, 18.00% women found it very poor while 8.33% reported as excellent. Only 22.33% women think that medicines are suitable for them. The cent percent women got treatment in primary health centre with fee. Out of them only 37.67% women advice PHC to other whereas 62.33% do not advise.

Table 4.57 reveals that women who were not utilising facilities of PHC have various reasons for it. 21.24% did not need it followed by 16.81% did not get suitable medicine, 11.95% found heavy rush in centre, 10.62% did not get free medicine, 6.19% due to unavailability of health worker, 5.75% feel that treatment is improper while 3.10% women prefer private hospital.

Table 4.58 reveals that sampled women have 228 children of age between 0 – 5 years in which 53.07% were male and 46.93% were female.

Table 4.59 reveals that all the cent percent of children were given bath just after delivery and all were given bath with hot water.

Table 4.56 : Details Opinion Regarding Working Status of Primary Health Center (PHC)

Number of women	*Easily reachable*		*Available medical facilities*		*Is wait done for long period*		*Is medicine distributed*		*Behavior of health workers or doctors of primary health centre (PHC)*	
	No	*Yes*	*No*	*Yes*	*No*	*Yes*	*No*	*Yes*	*Satisfied*	*Unsatisfied*
1	2	3	4	5	6	7	8	9	10	11
300	194	106	152	148	66	234	176	124	128	93
%	64.67%	35.33%	50.67%	49.33%	22.00%	78.00%	58.67%	41.33%	42.67%	31.00%

...Continued

Behavior of health workers or doctors of primary health center (PHC)		*Advised for medicine taken*		*Is these medicines suited*			*Available treatment*		*Do you advice primary health centre (PHC) to others*	
Excellent	*Very poor*	*No*	*Yes*	*No*	*Yes*	*Can't say*	*With fee*	*Free*	*No*	*Yes*
12	13	14	15	16	17	18	19	20	21	22
25	54	122	178	194	67	39	300	-	187	113
8.33%	18.00%	40.67%	59.33%	64.67%	22.33%	13.00%	100.00%	-	62.33%	37.67%

Table 4.57 : Reason for not Utilizing Services of Primary Health Center (PHC)

Number of women	*Number of women not utilising primary health centre (PHC)*	*Reasons*					
		Not needed	*Not situated on right place*	*Not open at right time*	*Low level of medical facilities*	*Heavy rash*	*Unavailability of health worker*
1	2	3	4	5	6	7	8
300	226	48	43	3	-	27	14
%	75.33%	21.24%	19.03%	1.33%	-	11.95%	6.19%

...Continued

Unavailability of free medicine	*Medicine not suited*	*Demand money for treatment*	*Improper treatment*	*Preference for private hospital*	*Others*	*No reply*
9	10	11	12	13	14	15
24	38	9	13	7	-	-
10.62%	16.81%	3.98%	5.75%	3.10%	-	-

Table 4.58 : Sex-wise Distribution of Number of Children between 0 - 5 Years of Age

Number of women	*Number of children*	*Male*	*Female*
300	228	121	107
%	100.00%	53.07%	46.93%

Table 4.59 : Bath Status of Newly Born Child

Number of children	*Bath after delivery*		
	No	*Yes*	
		By hot water	*By cold water*
228	-	228	-
%	-	100.00%	-

Table 4.60 reveals that out of all women 97.67% feed colostrums while 2.33% didn't feed due to their own illness.

Table 4.60 : Details of Colostrum Feeding to Children after Birth

Number of women respondent	*Colostrum feeding*			
	Yes	*Reasons for not feeding colostuim*		
		Thick	*Indigestible*	*Mother's illness*
300	293	-	-	7
%	97.67%	-	-	2.33%

Table 4.61 reveals that 84.21% respondent are advised for breast feeding where as 15.79% are not advised than 63.63% women are advised by female health worker, 13.40% by elderly ladies and 15.17% by private doctor.

Table 4.61 : Details of Advise given for Breast Feeding

Number of women	Number of women having children between the age of 0 - 5 years	Advise for breast feeding		Advise given by					
		No	Yes	Doc-tor	Private doctor	Nur-se	Elder lady	Female health worker	Others
300	209	33	124	-	9	-	17	98	-
%	69.67%	15.79%	84.21%	-	15.17%	-	13.40%	63.63%	-

Table 4.62 reveals that 32.06% women give first breast feeding to their baby after two hours of delivery followed by 29.67% after six hours than 14.09% after twelve hours, 9.09 after one day and 6.96% after two days.

Table 4.62 : Details of Timing of First Breast Feeding

Number of women	Number of women having children between the age of 0 - 5 years	Timing after birth					
		From birth	Two hours	Six hours	Twelve hours	One day	Two day
300	209	17	67	62	30	19	14
%	69.67%	8.13%	32.06%	29.67%	14.09%	9.09%	66.96%

Table 4.63 reveals that 35.53% children were presently breast feeding at the time of data collection while 64.47% were not.

Table 4.63 : Details of Presently Breast Feeding Children

Total number of children	Presently breast feeding	
	No	Yes
228	147	81
%	64.47%	35.53%

Table 4.64 reveals that out of the children between age 0 - 5 years 33.09% have feeded for nine months followed by 29.82% for eight months, 14.47% for ten months, 9.65% for seven months whereas only 1.32% were feeded for sixteen months.

Table 4.65 reveals that in the children of age 0 – 5 years. 32.46% have given semisolid food in sixth month followed by 28.95% in fifth month, 18.86% in fourth month, 16.67% in seventh month, 2.19% in eighth month and 0.88% in ninth month.

Table 4.66 reveals that out of the children between age 0 - 5 years of age 29.83% have given solid food first time in fifth month followed by 22.37% in seventh month, 14.04% in sixth month, 10.53% in ninth month and 0.44% in fifteenth month.

Table 4.67 reveals that in all, 69.67% women have children between 0 - 5 years of age. In which only 16.27% have knowledge and awareness about loose motion and only 3.88% have knowledge about pneumonia.

Table 4.68 reveals that in last six months 42.11% of 0 - 5 years age children were suffered with loose motion. Out of them 28.13% were treated in private hospital followed by 23.96% treated by household treatments than 22.92% by A.N.M. and 9.38% by government hospital while15.63% children are treated by other methods.

Table 4.64 : Details of Duration of Breast Feeding

Number of children	*Duration of breast feeding in months*					
	Four	*Five*	*Six*	*Seven*	*Eight*	*Nine*
228	6	14	17	22	68	74
%	2.63%	6.14%	7.46%	9.65%	29.82%	33.04%

...Continued

Ten	*Eleven*	*Twelve*	*Thirteen*	*Fourteen*	*Fifteen*	*Sixteen*	*Seventeen*
33	13	21	9	12	8	3	-
14.47%	5.70%	9.21%	3.95%	5.26%	3.51%	1.32%	-

Table 4.65 : Details of Age of Children for Giving Semisolid Food First Time

Number of children	Age of children in months										
	Four	Five	Six	Se-ven	Eight	Nine	Ten	Ele-ven	Twe-lve	Thir-teen	Four-teen
228	43	66	74	38	5	2	-	-	-	-	-
%	18.86%	28.95%	32.46%	16.67%	2.19%	0.88%	-	-	-	-	-

Table 4.66 : Details of Age of Children for Giving Solid Food First Time

Number of children	Age of children in months									
	Six	Seven	Eight	Nine	Ten	Ele-ven	Twe-lve	Thirt-een	Four-teen	Fift-een
228	32	51	68	24	14	13	11	9	5	1
%	14.04%	22.37%	29.83%	10.53%	6.14%	5.70%	4.82%	3.95%	2.19%	0.44%

Table 4.67 : Details of Information given by Health Women for Treatment of Loose Motion and Pneumonia

Number of women	Number of women having children between the age of 0 - 5 years	Awareness and knowledge provided by health workers			
		Loose motion		Pneumonia	
		No	Yes	No	Yes
300	209	175	34	201	8
%	69.67%	83.73%	16.27%	96.17%	3.83%

Table 4.68 : Details of suffered Children (under 5 year age) from Loose Motion in Last Six Months.

Total number of children	Suffered from loose motion		Treatment					
	No	Yes	Household treatment	ORS solution	Government hospital	Private hospital	Auxiliary nurse midwife (ANM)	Others
228	132	96	23		9	27	22	15
%	57.90%	42.11%	23.96%	-	9.38%	28.13%	22.92	15.63%

Table 4.69 reveals that women who have children between the age of 0 - 5 years were asked about identification of pneumonia. In which 29.67% reported increase in inhaling as a symptom of pneumonia followed by 24.40% difficulty in inhaling, 16.27% chest pain, 8.61% difficulty in drinking and 8.13% increase in cough, while 12.92% didn't reply the question.

Table 4.70 reveals that in last three years, 24.56% children were affected from Pneumonia. Out of them 62.50% were treated in private hospital followed by 33.93% in government hospital and 3.57% by household treatment.

Table 4.69 : Knowledge for Identification of Pneumonia

Number of women	Number of women having children between age of 0 - 5 years	Symptoms						No reply
		Difficulty in inhaling	Difficulty in drinking	Pain in chest	Increase in cough	Decline in health	Increase in inhaling	
300	209	51	18	34	17	-	62	27
%	67.67%	24.40%	8.61%	16.27%	8.13%	-	29.67%	12.92%

Table 4.70 : Details of Children Suffered from Pneumonia in Last Three Years

Number of children	Pneumonia suffers		Treatment by			
	Yes	No	Household treatment	Government hospital	Private hospital	Auxiliary nurse midwife (ANM)
228	56	172	2	19	35	-
100.00%	24.56%	75.44%	3.57%	33.93%	62.50%	-

Table 4.71 reveals that 80.38% children have received vaccination card while 19.62% haven't.

Table 4.71 : Details of Vaccination Card

Number of women	Number of women having children between the age of 0 - 5 years	Is vaccination card provided	
		No	Yes
300	209	41	168
%	69.67%	19.62%	80.38%

Table 4.72 reveals that in all, 37.72% children were vaccinated for diphtheria, 85.09% were vaccinated for polio,

53.07% were vaccinated for tetanus and 28.51% were vaccinated for small pox.

Table 4.72 : Details of Vaccination Status among the Children

Number of children	*Diphtheria*		*Polio*		*Tetanus*		*Smallpox*	
	No	*Yes*	*No*	*Yes*	*No*	*Yes*	*No*	*Yes*
228	142	86	34	194	107	121	163	65
%	62.28%	37.72%	14.91%	85.09%	46.93%	53.07%	71.49%	28.51%

Table 4.73 reveals various reasons for not vaccinating their children's. It is observed from the table that unawareness about place of vaccination is most frequent reason i.e., in 40.85% cases of diphtheria, in 29.41% cases of polio, in 59.81% cases of tetanus and in 46.63% cases of smallpox. Less age of children is another reason i.e., in 23.94% cases of diphtheria, in 35.29% cases of polio, in 21.49% cases of tetanus and in 17.18% cases of smallpox while some respondents did not believe in vaccination i.e., in 7.04% cases of diphtheria, in 11.76% cases of polio, in 5.61% cases of tetanus and in 14.11% cases of smallpox. For some respondent place of vaccination was not in reach i.e., in 8.45% cases of diphtheria, in 17.65% cases of polio, in 4.67% cases of tetanus and in 3.68% cases of smallpox.

Table 4.74 reveals that in most of the cases last vaccination of children between 0 - 5 years age conducted at aganwadi (56.14%) followed by 17.11% in school, 2.63% by female health worker and 0.88% at P.H.C.

Table 4.73 : Reasons for not Vaccinating Children

Vaccination	*Number of unvaccinated children*	*Less age of children*	*Unawareness about place of vaccination*	*Unawareness about importance of vaccination*	*Side effects of vaccination*	*Unawareness about time of vaccination*	*Do not believe in vaccination*
1	2	3	4	5	6	7	8
Diphtheria	142	34	58	14	-	-	10
%	100.00%	23.94%	40.85%	9.86%	-	-	7.04%
Polio	34	12	10	-	-	-	4
%	100.00%	35.29%	29.41%	-	-	-	11.76%
Tetanus	107	23	64	9	-	-	6
%	100.00%	21.49%	59.81%	8.41%	-	-	5.61%
Smallpox	163	28	76	15	-	-	23
%	100.00%	17.18%	46.63%	9.20%	-	-	14.11%

....continued

Place of vaccination is faraway	*Unsuitable time of vaccination*	*Unavailability of vaccination health worker*	*Unavailability of vaccine*	*Busy schedule of mother*	*Illness of mother*	*Illness of child*	*Children were not vaccinated by health worker do to their illness*
9	10	11	12	13	14	15	16
12	9	-	-	-	5	-	-
8.45%	6.34%	-	-	-	3.52%	-	-
6	-	-	-	-	2	-	-
17.65%	-	-	-	-	5.88%	-	-
5	-	-	-	-	-	-	-
4.67%	-	-	-	-	-	-	-
6	-	-	-	-	7	-	8
3.68%	-	-	-	-	4.29%	-	4.91%

Table 4.74 : Place of Last Vaccination

Number of children	Place of last vaccination								Not vaccinated
	Government hospital	Primary health center (PHC)	Female health worker	Private hospital	Private doctor	Aganwadi	Sch-ool	Not known	
228	-	2	6	-	-	128	39	19	34
%	-	0.88%	2.63%	-	-	56.14%	17.11%	8.33%	14.91%

Table 4.75 reveals that in all, 29.82% children were given vitamin A solution while 10.53% didn't are known about it. Out of 29.82% children 79.41% were given vitamin A solution once followed by 11.76% twice and 8.82% thrice.

Table 4.75 : Details of Frequency of received Vitamin - A Solution by the Children

Number of children	Vitamin - A			Repetition				
	No	Yes	Not know	Once	Twice	Thrice	Fourth	Not remember
228	136	68	24	54	8	6	-	-
%	59.65%	29.82%	10.53%	79.41%	11.76%	8.82%	-	-

Table 4.76 reveals that in all, 33.33% children have given iron and folic acid tablets in which 57.89% were given once followed by 25.00% twice, 10.53% thrice while 6.58% not remembered the repeated number.

Table 4.76 : Distribution of Iron & Folic Acid Tablets

Number of children	*Utilized*		*Repetition*				
	No	*Yes*	*Once*	*Twice*	*Thrice*	*Fourth*	*Not remember*
228	152	76	44	19	8	-	5
%	66.67%	33.33%	57.89%	25.00%	10.53%	-	6.58%

5
Conclusions

Tribal groups of India widely varying ecological and geoclimatic condition in different concentration throughout the country as a 8.08% of the total population (Census, 1991) and are distinct biological isolated with characteristic cultural and socio-economic set up. The health status of these tribal population groups is as such a function of the interaction between their socio-cultural and socio-biological practices, genetic attributes and the environmental condition. They widely varying prevalent health practices, use of indigenous herbal drugs, taboos and superstition are also responsible for determining the health behaviour practices of the tribal groups which have a compounding effect on health status including fertility, mortality and morbidity patterns. India has become a signatory to the Alma Ata Declaration in 1978, committing itself to achieve "Health for All" by the year 2000. In National Health Policy (NHP) scheduled tribes and scheduled castes become priority groups for providing better health care services. The current strategies and programmes for implementing the National Health Policy through integrated health programmes will include the following reinforcing components (1) Improvement of environmental sanitation (2) Immunisation (3) Family planning (4) Nutrition (5) Health education.

There are about 538 scheduled tribal population groups in the country (People of India, 1994) existing at various phases of development. Most of the tribal groups are residing in interior, remote inaccessible areas with various types of health hazards and lack of modern health care facilities. Some of them living in the remote area following hunting and food gathering etc.

A critical review clearly indicate that hardly and holistic study carried out among the tribal population on the nature of fertility - mortality (abortions, still births) in relation to interaction between socio-cultural and biological parameters especially in Madhya Pradesh tribal groups. Such data are important for planning of effective need based, area and group specific health care strategies in these groups, where the available reports revealed that they tend to under utilise the available health care facilities. So each tribe has to be studied carefully so as to develop effective health care measures. Keeping this in view embodied study has been carried among the Raj Gonds of Sagar district, Madhya Pradesh. The objectives of present study are:

- To investigate the maternal and child mortality and morbidity patterns and associated factors.
- To elicit their Knowledge Attitudes and Practices (KAP) regarding Reproductive and Child Health (RCH) problems.

The Raj Gond is tribal sub-division of Gond, which belongs to dravidian family. According to Gonds Forsyth the Raj Gonds are in many cases the descendents of alliances between Rajput adventures and Gonds. The Raj Gond rank with the Hindu cultivating castes and Brahmins take water from them. The main occupation of Raj Gonds is cultivation and labour. According to 1981 census the tribal population of Gond in the Madhya Pradesh was 3,770,000 persons in which about 63864 (comprising **10359** eligible couples aged between 15 - 49 years according to population progression method) resides in Sagar District.

The concern data has been collected from Raj Gond predominated inhabited villages of Kelsi, Kehli and Sagar blocks of Sagar district in which more than 70% of this population resides. In sampling frame, the villages of these blocks having Raj Gond were arranged in descending order on the basis of their population. The village having greater concentration was selected by probability proportion. By this method twenty five villages namely Apchand, Barpani, Dhura, Padariya, Bada Piperiya (Sagar block) Kadta, Jamuniya, Sahajpur, Kalan, Semra Gond, Tada, Datpura, Murga, Padasiya (Rehli block) and Chauka, Ghana, Tumri, Jamunia, Ramgarha, Jamuniya near Chauka, Kachhaua, Anghori Duhli, Nandiya (Kesli block) has been selected. From these villages different samples were taken but the sample size of each village under study has vary on the basis of their population in order to make the sample a representative one. For the present investigation 300 genetically unrelated couples (comprising males and females) which cover 2.8% of the total eligible couples were investigated for the reproductive and child health informations with the help of genealogy enumerating pregnancy to pregnancy with suitable cross checks by using structured schedule, observations, case study method. The data has been analysed with the help of statistical parameters such as percentage, mean, standard deviation, by using SPSS package. The findings of the study are given below:

1. The 80.67% women and 56.33% men cannot read and write whereas 19.33% women and 43.66% men can.
2. Most of the women have two children (29.33%) followed by one (28.00%), five (10.67%), three (10.00%), four (9.33%), six (7.67%), seven (3.00%) and eight (2.00%).
3. Out of total pregnancies, live births are most frequent (93.82%) followed by abortions (6.17%), still births

(12.73%), child death (9.00%) and juvenile death (5.64%), Infant death rate is found highest (13.55) than child death rate (9.59), adolescent death rate (6.01) and reproductive wastage (6.17).

4. The 16.33% women respondents have faced abortions in which all the cent percent abortions were self abortions. Out of them 49.25% women were aborted once followed by 20.89% twice and 2.98% thrice.

5. Out of the women who faced abortions, 38.76% suffered from excess bleeding with in one week after abortion followed by 10.20% from high fever and 2.04% from fouls smelling while 48.98% have all problems.

6. Women have self abortion have been asked about health care consultation, out of them 77.55% didn't take any consultation or treatment after abortion while 4.08% women have consulted with health worker or primary health centre or elder ladies, rest of the 10.20% women went to private doctor for their problems.

7. Women who faced still births are 3.67%, out of which 21.43% cases were found in fifth pregnancy followed by 14.28% in second, fourth, seventh and eighth rest of 7.14% case were found in third and sixth pregnancy.

8. In last seven years (1996 - 2002) 95.33% women become pregnant. Total 343 pregnancies were known in this period. 19.00% women become twice in these years. Highest frequency of pregnancies 19.53% is found in year 2000 followed by 17.20% in year 2001, 16.32% in year 1999 while lowest frequency is observed 6.70% in year 2002.

9. Only 34.00% women respondents were visited by Auxiliary nurse midwife (ANM) during pregnancy while 66.00% were not visited.

10. Out of these 34.00% women visited of Auxiliary nurse midwife (ANM) maximum 25.49% women were visited in seventh month followed by 22.55% in eight and fourth month respectively and six month (13.72%), while only 2.94% were visited in third month of pregnancy.

11. Only 4.67% women respondent were advised for health checkup by Auxiliary nurse midwife (A.N.M.) while 89.33% were not advised and rest of 6.00% have forgotten about it.

12. During pregnancy no women did not use sex identification techniques for identify sex of a baby in her womb.

13. During pregnancy only 12.00% took their body weight, only 7.33% went for blood pressure checkup and only 34.00% have taken iron and folic acid tablets.

14. Out of 34.00% women who took iron and folic acid tablets 50.98% women were advised and given two tablets for a day followed by 37.25% one tablet and 3.92% three tablet whereas 7.84% women did not remember the number of tablets per day.

15. Only 14.33% women have received tetanus toxied injection during pregnancy where as 85.66% have not received..

16. Out of these 14.33% women 90.69 % have given one tetanus toxied injection while 9.30% have given two.

17. During pregnancy respondent women have faced various health problems. Swollen in hand and feet is found most frequent (35.33%) followed by weakness (14.00%), tiredness (11.33%), heaviness (7.66%) not feeling well (6.667%), eye problem (1.33%), bleeding (1.00%) and no sensation of embryo movement (0.33%), whereas 5.33% women faced other problems,

15.33% faced more than one problem and 2.66% did not reply the question.

18. During pregnancy 17.67% women have utilized health care services whereas 71.00% did not utilize and 11.33% women did not face any problem.

19. Out of 17.67% women who took treatment for problems during pregnancy, 50.94% have visited to private doctor followed by 28.30% health workers and 20.75% government doctors.

20. During pregnancy only 1.33% women were advised for regular health checkup by health workers.

21. The 75.33% have paid government fee for health checkup while 24.67% have got free checkup.

22. Most of the deliveries i.e., 94.33% were conducted at home with the help of elder ladies followed by 4.00% at Primary health center and 1.66% at District hospital.

23. Delivery instruments were not available in 94.33% cases while in 5.67% cases instruments were available.

24. During delivery only 26.33% women have suffered with various health problems. Pain before delivery is most frequent problem reported by 60.76% followed by pains with short intervals of time by 15.19%, not feeling well by 11.39% and pains of longer duration by 8.86% women.

25. In 82.67% deliveries new blade has been used as a tool for cutting navel cord followed by old blades in 8.00% and knife in 3.67% cases while in 5.67% cases other instruments have been used. Out of these in only 12.67% cases the tool has been boiled before using where as in 82.00% it has been used without boiled and 5.33% women didn't reply this question.

26. After one week of delivery 75.67% women have suffered with various health problems. Out of these health problem back pain in 23.79% respondents is most frequent followed by headache 17.18%, high fever 16.74% while foul smelling is least frequent in 1.32% women.

27. Out of 75.67% women who have faced health problems after delivery only 23.55% have utilise treatment facilities while 76.65% did not take treatment 50.94% treated women consulted private doctors followed by 28.80% Auxiliary nurse midwife (ANM) and 20.75% and government doctor.

28. Only 32.67% women have various reproductive health problems. Out of them burning sensation in urinal is most frequent problem by 47.96% women and 12.24% suffering with vaginal secretion. Secretion type is thin white or thick brown white in 16.67% cases while thick white in 8.33% cases. In women suffering with vaginal secretion 23.47% have back pain and 15.30% have fever due to secretion. Other health problem with buring sensation in vagina are found in 9.18% case and pain during intercourse in 8.16% cases.

29. Out of 32.62% women having reproductive health problems, 32.65% have conversation with their husband followed by 23.47% women with mother or mother in law, 9.18% with elderly ladies. A large number of women i.e., 24.98% don't share their problem with any one due of hesitation.

30. Out of 32.62% women who reproductive health problems, 28.57% have consultation with private doctor 28.57% followed by 23.46% with Auxiliary nurse midwife (A.N.M.) while 18.37% do not take any treatment for problems and 3.06% utilise traditional treatment.

31. Out of total respondent 37.67% women have knowledge about Acquired immune deficiency syndrome (AIDS) and 5.33% women did not reply. Out of these aware women 37.17% get this knowledge through radio followed by 30.09% by husband, 14.15% by friends, 11.50% by television and 3.54% by *dais*.

32. Out of these 37.67% women those are aware to AIDS, 25.66% think that heterosexuality is the mode of transmission of AIDS. According to 21.24% women intercourse and 5.30% kissing can transmitted AIDS while 10.62% women knows that unhygienic activities can transmit it followed by 15.92% sleeping with infected person and 7.96% by the use of others used needle.

33. Out of the women who are for AIDS 27.43% know that AIDS can be prevent, but 42.48% do not know about medium of is prevention while condom is the preventive medium for 23.53% women followed by safe intercourse for 8.82% women and blood test before donation for 5.88% women whereas 61.76% answered all these medium.

34. Only 29.33% women are aware to sexually transmitted diseases while 5.34% women didn't reply the question. Women those are aware, out of them 21.59% got information by their husbands followed by 19.31% from radio and 13.64% by health workers or friends.

35. A large percentage of women i.e., 64.67% is aware about malaria. Out of them husband is the source of knowledge in 24.74% cases followed by radio in 23.71% cases and malaria workers in 16.49% cases.

36. Out of these respondents 16.00% women were pregnant at the time of data collection.

37. According to 61.00% women childbirth can be limited and 39.00% thinks that it is not possible. In 61.00% women, for 33.88% condom is the best medium to limit child birth followed by 19.67% reported oral pills than 15.84% sterilisation while 30.60% all these methods.

38. At the time data collection 49.33% respondents were using family welfare device. Out of them in 42.57% cases husbands and in 26.35% cases wives were using devices while in 31.08% cases both husbands and wives were using family welfare device.

39. Out of these 49.33% respondents using family welfare device, 64.19% were using condom followed by 14.18% tubectomy, 12.16% oral pills, 8.10% safe period and 1.35% vasectomy method.

40. Women who have information about family welfare devices are 61.00%. For 36.06% of them husband was the source of information followed by 26.23% radio, 15.30% A.N.M., 13.11% friends and 9.29% television.

41. Out of these 49.33% respondents using family welfare device 21.62% women were facing health problems due to use of family welfare device. Body or back pain is most frequent reported by 59.37% women followed by 18.76% reported vomiting sensation than 12.50% fattiness, 6.25% heaviness and 3.12% irregular menstrual cycle.

42. Women who health problems due to use of family welfare device were 21.62% of presently users. Out of them 34.38% have taken treatment, 81.82% women get treatment from private doctor while 18.18% from government doctor.

43. Out of these 49.33% women 58.11% were not satisfied with the family welfare devices they were using while 41.89% were satisfied.

44. The place chosen for tubectomy was camp by 10.18% women while 4.72% women were sterilisation in primary health centre. At the time of data collection 49.33% women were using family welfare devices. For 69.59% of them devices are easily available from female health worker and for 3.38% these are not available easily on shop while 16.22% women did not answer the question.

45. Out of these 50.67% respondent who were not using family welfare devices at the time of data collection only 34.87% have used them in past. In 43.40% cases device was used by husband while in 33.96% cases it was used by wives. 43.40% couples used condoms followed by 33.96% used oral pills and 22.64% used safe period. In these women 35.53% were presently not using due to unsatisfation followed by 27.63% unsatisfation by devices, 11.84% expecting children & 8.55% due to body or back pain, while 1.97% were not utilising device due to difficulty in use and 1.32% due to irregular menstrual cycle.

46. Out of these 50.67% respondent not using any family welfare devices at the time of data collection and only 24.34% respondent devices were distributed by health worker while 75.66% did not get these devices.

47. According to 61.00% of total respondent family welfare device are easily available while 17.67% didn't have information about its availability and 21.33% said that devices are not available.

48. Out of total respondent 57.33% were interested in utilising family welfare device. 45.35% were choose condom followed by 31.40% tubectomy, 12.21% safe period, 9.88% oral pills and 1.16% vasectomy.

49. Out of 50.67% women not using any family welfare devices. 23.03% were not using it because they don't

like to use it followed by 15.13% due to unawareness, 9.21% thinks it is antireligious 8.55% feared about power loss, 3.95% because of husband's opposition and 1.32% due to family opposition.

50. For 42.00% respondent head of the family is the decision maker for sterilisation followed by husband in 32.97% cases, herself in 8.00% cases, and in 2.00% case mother-in-law while 13.67% women did not answer the question.

51. The 41.33% respondents were agreed for tubectomy whereas 58.67% were not.

52. Health worker have visited 44.67% respondents in last three months while 48.33% were not visited and 7.00% did not remember. In 58.21% cases visits were taken by *aganwadi* worker rest of 41.79% by doctor. Out of 44.67% women who were visited by health worker 64.93% were satisfied with their visits.

53. Primary health centre was utilising by 24.67% women and only 37.84% were satisfied with the treatment facilities of centre while 62.16% were unsatisfied.

54. Primary health centre is easily reachable for 35.33% women while not approachable for 64.67% women. According to 49.33% women medical facilities are available in primary health centre. 78.00% women thinks that they have to wait for a long time in PHC. According to 41.33% women medicines are distributed in PHC. Behaviour of health workers and doctors of P.H.C. was satisfactory for 42.6% women while it is unsatisfactory for 31.00% women, 18.00% women found it very poor while 8.33% reported as excellent. Only 22.33% women think that medicines are suitable for them. The cent percent women got treatment in primary health centre with fee. Out of them only 37.67% women advice PHC to other whereas 62.33%

do not advise.

55. Women who were not utilising facilities of PHC have various reasons for it. 21.24% did not need it followed by 16.81% did not get suitable medicine, 11.95% found heavy rush in centre, 10.62% did not get free medicine, 6.19% due to unavailability of health worker, 5.75% feel that treatment is improper while 3.10% women prefer private hospital.

56. In all women have 228 children of age between 0 - 5 years in which 53.07% were male and 46.93% were female.

57. All the cent percent of children were given bath just after delivery and all were given bath with hot water.

58. Out of all women 97.67% feed colostrums while 2.333% didn't feed due to their own illness.

59. In the children between age 0 - 5 years 35.53% were feeding at the time of data collection while 64.47% were not.

60. Out of the children between age 0 - 5 years 33.09% have feeded for nine months followed by 29.82% for eight months, 14.47% for ten months, 9.65% for seven months whereas only 1.32% were feeded for sixteen months.

61. In the children of age 0 - 5 years 32.46% have given semisolid food in sixth month followed by 28.95% in fifth month, 18.86% in fourth month, 16.67% in seventh month, 2.19% in eighth month and 0.88% in ninth month.

62. Out of the children between age 0 - 5 years of age 29.83% have given solid food first time in fifth month followed by 22.37% in seventh month, 14.04% in sixth month, 10.53% in ninth month and 0.44% in fifteenth month.

63. In all the women 69.67% have children of 0 - 5 years of age. In which only 16.27% have knowledge and awareness about loose motion and only 3.88% have knowledge about pneumonia.

64. In last six months 42.11% of 0 - 5 years age children were suffered with loose motion. Out of them 28.13% were treated in private hospital followed by 23.96% treated by household treatments than 22.92% by A.N.M. and 9.38% by government hospital while15.63% children are treated by other methods.

65. Women who have children between the age of 0 - 5 years were asked about identification of pneumonia. In which 29.67% reported increase in inhaling as a symptom of pneumonia followed by 24.40% difficulty in inhaling, 16.27% chest pain, 8.61% difficulty in drinking and 8.13% increase in cough, while 12.92% didn't reply the question.

66. In last three years 24.56% children were affected from Pneumonia. Out of them 62.50% were treated in private hospital followed by 33.93% in government hospital and 3.57% by household treatment.

67. The 80.38% children have received vaccination card while 19.62% haven't.

68. In all children 37.72% were vaccinated for diphtheria, 85.09% were vaccinated for polio, 53.07% were vaccinated for tetanus and 28.51% were vaccinated for small pox.

69. Various reasons for not vaccinating children are found in which unawareness about place of vaccination is most frequent *i.e.,* in 40.85% cases of diphtheria, in 29.41% cases of polio, in 59.81% cases of tetanus and in 46.63% cases of smallpox. Less age of children is another reason *i.e.,* in 23.94% cases of diphtheria, in

35.29% cases of polio, in 21.49% cases of tetanus and in 17.18% cases of smallpox while some respondents did not believe in vaccination *i.e.*, in 7.04% cases of diphtheria, in 11.76% cases of polio, in 5.61% cases of tetanus and in 14.11% cases of smallpox. For some respondent place of vaccination was not in reach *i.e.*, in 8.45% cases of diphtheria, in 17.65% cases of polio, in 4.67% cases of tetanus and in 3.68% cases of smallpox.

70. Last vaccination of children between 0 - 5 years age conducted at *aganwadi* in 56.14% cases followed by 17.11% in school, 2.63% by female health worker and 0.88% at P.H.C.

71. In all children 29.82% were given vitamin A solution while 10.53% didn't are known about it. Out of 29.82% children 79.41% were given vitamin A solution once followed by 11.76% twice and 8.82% thrice.

72. In all children 33.33% children have given iron and folic acid tablets in which 57.89% were given once followed by 25.00% twice, 10.53% thrice while 6.58% not remembered the repeated number.

In all health facilities prevails among Raj Gonds. This information will be helpful in understanding of genetico-environmental interaction at according reproductive mechanism for the formulation of need based health care policy in the tribal population to uplift their health standards.

Bibliography

Abou Zahr, C. and Wardlaw, T. 2001. Matrernal mortality at the end of decade: Signs of progress. *Bulletin of World Health Organization*, 79(**6**): 561-568.

Agarwal, D. 2001. Reprodutive tract infections: Challenges and responses. *Health for the Millions*, 27(**3**): 21-23.

Ahmed, S.H. 1973. Maternal Health, Child Health and Family Planning: A Plea for Integration Approach. *Indian Paediatrics*, 10(**1**): 13-17.

Alwani, C.M. 1976. Social Aspect of Family Planning. *Journal of Obstetrics and Gynaecology of India*, 26(**1**): 24-28.

Arora, A. and Choudhary, A. 1993. Health Modernity in Rural Tribal of Chotanagpur and Santhal Pargana. *Social Change*, 23(**1**):43-55.

Ascadi, G.T. F. and Ascadi, J. 1990. Safe Motherhood in South Asia : Sociocultural and demographic aspects of maternal health, Background paper prepared for the *Safe Motherhood South Asia Conference*, Lahore.

Bajpai, S. 2001. Indian system of medicine in reproductive and child health. *Health for the Millions*, 27(**3**): 16-18.

Balakrishna, S. 1971. *Family Planning Knowledge, Attitude and Practice: A Sample Survey in Andhra Pradesh*. Research Report, National Institute of Community Development, Hyderabad.

Basu, S.K., Jindal, A. 1990. *Genetic and Socio-cultural Determinants of Tribal Health: A Primitive Kutia Kondhs of Tribal Group of Phulbani District, Orissa.* Research Report, NIHFW, New Delhi.

Basu, S.K., Jindal, A. and Kshatriya, G.K. 1990. The determinants of health seeking behavior among tribal population of Bastar district, M.P. *South Asian Anthropologist,* 11(**1**): 1-6.

BCC. CINI, SEWA-Rural and Streehitkarini, 1997. Prevalence of clinically detectable gynecological morbidity in India: Results from four community based studies. *Journal of Family Welfare,* 43(**4**): 8-16.

Begum, S., Arokiasamy, P. and Acharya, R. 1998. Factors affecting complications during delivery: An analysis of NHFS data. *Journal of Family Welfare,* 44(**1**): 15-26.

Begum. Z. and Nurul Islam, M. 2001. Factor affecting utilization of MCH services in Bangladesh. *Journal of Family welfare,* 47(**1**): 68-78.

Bhandari, B.S. 1989. Under-Utilization of MCH Services: The major factors for very high IMR in rural Rajasthan. *Indian Paediatrics,* 26 (**2**): 111-117.

Bharati, Premananda and Basu, A. 1990. Fertility mortality and maternal anemic status in a village population of West Bengal, India, *Annals of Human Biology,* **17**: 331-342.

Bhargawa, I. 1983. Integrated approach to Maternal and Child Health and Family Planning. *Indian Paediatrics,* 20 (**1**): 38-44.

Bhatia, J.C. and Neumann, A.K. 1980. Inter-Spousal communication and practice of contraception in India. *Journal of Family Welfare,* 26(**2**): 53-62.

Bhatia, J.C. and Cleland, J. 1994. Self Reported symptoms

of gynecological morbidity and their treatment in South India. *Studies in Family Planning*, 26(**4**): 203-216.

Bhatt Mari, P.N., Navaneetham, K., and Irudaya Rajan, S. 1992. *Maternal Mortality in India: Estimates from an Econometric Model*. Population Research Center, Dharwad.

Bhattacharya, M., Singh, G., Banerjee, S.C. and Narula, R.K. 1993. An indepth analysis of women with post-abortal bleeding. *Journal of Family Welfare*, 39(**2**):17-21.

Bir, T. 2001. *Dynamics of Health Culture: Urban Slum Community and Behaviour*, Rajat Publications, New Delhi.

Caldwell, J.C. 1982. *Theory of Fertility Decline*. Academic Press, New York.

Caldwell, J.C. 1986. Routes of low mortality in poor countries. *Population and Development Review*, **12**.

Census of India 1981. *Special Tables for Scheduled Tribes*, Series - II, Madhya Pradesh Part IX, Registrar General and Census Commissioner of India, New Delhi.

Census of India 1991. Office of Registrar General and Census Commissioner of India, New Delhi.

Chandra, P. 2001. Child health development fter Alma Ata Declaration. *Indian Pediatrics*, 38(**17**): 1129-1143.

Chatterjee, G. 2000. *Health Nutrition and Diseases*, Rajat Publications, New Delhi.

Chopra, K. 1999. Tribal Health (In) *Health and Family Welfare Development in Independent India*. NIHFW, New Delhi, 247-258.

Das. N. 1972. Factors related to knowledge, family size preference and practices of family planning in India. *Journal of Family Welfare*, 19(**1**): 1-8.

Datta, K.K. 1980. Morbidity pattern amongst rural pregnant women in Alwar, Rajasthan: A cohort study. *Health and Population: Perspectives and Issues,* 3(**4**): 282-292.

Devi, B. 1972. Knowledge and attitudes to family planning among the Kuvi-Kandha. *Journal of Family Welfare,* 19(**2**): 41-46.

Dutta, R. 1973. Public health and family planning : A study of Inter-relationship in India. *American Journal of Public Health,* 63(**2**): 128-135.

Dwivedi, P. 2003. *Demographic Profile and Health Care Practices among the Baigas of Samnapur Block of Dindori District, Madhya Pradesh.* M.Sc. Dissertation, Dr. Hari Singh Gour University, Sagar, Madhya Pradesh. (Unpublished)

Ghosh, B.N. and Mukherjee, A.B. 1989. An analysis of health services coverage of a primary health center in West Bengal. *Indian Journal of Paediatrics, 48*(**1**): 9-18

Government of Madhya Pradesh. 1993. *Survey of Causes of Death (Rural).* Department of Economics and Statistics, Bhopal. 1996.

Gulati, B. 1971. *Integration of Family Planning with Maternity and Child Health Services in Council for Social Development: Aspects of Population Policy in India.* Council for Social Development. New Delhi.

Gupta, K. 2001. Fertility and contraceptive prevalence in India: Glimpses form NFHS II. *Health for the Millions,* 27(**3**): 13-15.

Gupta, R.B.1991 Assess to basic services to women and children in urban slums. *Proceedings of the Workshop on Improving Young Women's Health and Development,* ICMR, New Delhi.

Hutter, I. 1994. *Being Pregnant in Rural South India,* PDOD publications.

Jain, A. 2000. *The study of Maternal and Child Health Practices Among Seminomadic Lohar Gadiyas of Malthone Block of Sagar District, Madhya Pradesh.* M.Sc. Dissertation, Dr. Hari Singh Gour University, Sagar, Madhya Pradesh. (Unpublished)

Jaiswal, M. 1985. Health Modernity and its correlates in women of South Bihar. *Social Change,* 15(**2**): 7-14.

Jaiswal, M. and Singh, A.K. 1989. Health Modernity in the Tribals of South Bihar. *Social Change,* 19(**1**): 13-29.

Jacobson, J. 1993. "Women's reproductive health: The Silent emergency", *World Watch Paper,* **102**, World Watch Institute, Washington, D.C.

Jha, S. 1983. Indian women's health status in the context of social development. *Journal of Family Welfare,* 29(**1**): 19-25.

Jorapur, P.B. 1979. *Problems in Implementing Family Planning Programmes.* A study of medical and para-medical personnel, Nutrition, Health and Family Planning in Karnataka. A study of ICDS, Ph.D. Thesis, Unpublished, S.V. University, Tirupati.

Kale, B.D. 1966. *Family Planning Enquiry in Dharwar Town.* Institute of Economic Research, Vidyagiri. Research Report, Demographic Research Center. Dharwar.

Kanitkar, T. and Sinha, R.K. 1989. Antenatal Care Services in Five States of India. (In) *Population Transition in India.* Volume 2, (Eds), by S.N. Singh, M.K. Premi, P.S. Bhatia and A. Bose, B.R. Publication, New Delhi.

Kaul, P. 1991. Utilization of maternal and child health services in rural areas of Jammu and Kashmir. *Nursing journal of India,* 82(**1**): 9-16.

Kaur, G. and Singh, T.R. 1982. Acceptance of family planning practices among rural women. *Indian Journal of Public Health*, 26(**3**): 185-192.

Khan, M.E. and Rao, S. 1989. Do welfare services reach couples below the poverty line ? A case study of family welfare programme in Bihar. (In) *Population Transition in India*, Volume 2, (Eds) by S.N. Singh, M.K. Premi, P.S. Bhatia and A. Bose, B.R. Publication, New Delhi.

Khan, M.E. 1985. Access to Health and Family Planning Services in Rural Uttar Pradesh : A Micro Level Evaluation. *Studies in Population Health and Family Planning Research Group*, **47**.

Knowless, S. 1987. Spontenous abortion and the pathology of early pregnancy. (In) *Fetal and Neonatal Pathology*, (Ed) by J.W. Keeling, Springer, Verlag.

Kohli, B.R. and Goel, O.P., 1974. *Factors Associated with Knowledge and Practices of Family Planning*. National Institute of Family Planning, New Delhi. Technical Paper No. 19.

Koteshwar, R.K. 1970. *Seven Years of Family Planning in Dharwar: A Study of Knowledge, Attitude and Practice of Family Planning*. Research Report, Demographic Research Center.Dharwar.

Kumar, A. 1982. Utilization Pattern of MCH Services in an Urban Community, *Newsletter*, 8(**2**): 55-60.

Mahadevan, K. 1983. *Diffusion of Family .Planning Innovations Through Satisfied Adopters: A Strategy for Programme Development*. Paper Presented at Indian Science Congress, Association, Tirupati.

Maitra, N., Baxi, R.K. and Hazra, M. 1994. Adolescent sexuality, education and sources of information. *Indian Journal of Maternal and Child Health*, **5**: 95-98.

Malhotra, A.K. 1988. Assessment of efficacy of BCC vaccination among slum children of Agra city. *Indian Journal of Public Health*, 32 (**1**): 21-26.

Mamgain, M.C. 1972. MCH and Family Planning in *Proceedings of the International Conference of Family Planning*, (Ed) P.C. Bhatla, Indian Medical Association, New Delhi.

Mandakini, K. 1971. *Utilization of Social and Welfare Services in Greater Bombay*. Tata Institute of Social Sciences, Bombay, Series: **34**.

Mouli, A.S.C. and Mouli, S. 1981. Adopters and Non-adopters of Family Planning in Indian Villages: A case study, *The Journal of Family Welfare*, 27(**3**): 23-25.

Mukherjee, B.N. 1975. Status of women as related to family planning. *Journal of Population Research*, 2(**1**): 23-28.

Murali, A. and Kotaria, M. 1980. Perception regarding need for antenatal care among rural and urban women in Delhi. *Indian Journal of Public Health*, 24(**2**): 73-79.

Murthy, J.S. and Ramesh 1978. Selection Intercity among the tribal population of Adhilabad district. *Social Biology*, **25**: 302-305.

Nag, M. 1983. Impact of Social and Economic Development on Mortality. Comparative study of Kerala and West Bengal. *Economic and Political Weekly*, **22**.

National Family Health Survey, 1992-93. *MCH and Family Planning*. International Institute of population Sciences, Bombay, August 1995.

ORG, 1974. *Family Planning Practices in India: The First All India Survey Report*. Operation Research Group, Baroda.

Pandey, G.D. 1999. *A Study of Effect of Social Factors on Human Fertility and Family Planning with Special*

Reference to Major Primitive. Tribes of Madhya Pradesh. D.Litt. Dissertation in Sociology, Rani Durgawati Vishwavidayalaya, Jabalpur. (Unpublished)

Pandey, G.D. Roy and Tiwary A. 1996. Socio-cultural characteristics and health seeking behaviour of khairwars of M.P. *Journal of Family Welfare,* 42(**2**): 45-49.

Pandey, G.D. and Tiwary, R.S. 1993. Socio-cultural characteristics and health seeking behavior of the Hill Korwa, *Journal of Family Welfare,* 39(**2**): 44-48.

Parchure, N. and Warvadekar, J. 2004. Awareness of RTI, STI and HIV-AIDS in Madhya Pradesh. Paper presented in *National Seminar on Reproductive and Child Health Problem in Rural Area of India.* Organized by Department of Anthropology, Dr. Hari Singh Gour University, Sagar (M.P.)

Parker, R.L. and Wolff, M.C. 1984. The impact of health services on Family Planning Practices. Paper presented at the *11th Annual International Health Conference,* Arlington, Virginia.

Paruthi, R. and Gupta, M.C. 2001. Reproductive and child health: Role of health promotion and education under the revised Paradigm. Health Education in South East Asia, 16(**1**): 18-35.

Pathak, K.B. and Singh, B.S. 1993. Adolescent Motherhood and Maternal Mortality in India, (In) *Dynamics of Population and Family Welfare* (Eds), K.B. Pathak, U.P. Sinha and A.. Pandey, Himalaya Publishing House,Bombay.

Pathak, K.B. and Ram, F. 1993. Adolescent Motherhood Problems and Consequences. *Journal of Family Welfare,* 39(**1**): 17-23.

Pawar, R.G. 1983. Utilization of preventive services: An elaborative study of vaccine acceptors. *Indian Journal of Preventive and Social Medicine,* 14 (**1&2**): 33-40.

Pethe, V.P. 1962. Practice of contraception and attitudes towards family planning. Finding of a sample survey. *AICC Economic Review.*

Poddar, A.K. 1988. A coparative study on the immunization status of children and mothers between rural and urban areas. *Indian Journal of Public Health,* 32(**2**): 55-62.

Prasad, C.V.S. and Somayajulu, U.V. 1992. A comparative study of the accessibility of health and family welfare services among slum dwellers. *Journal of Family Welfare,* 38(**1**) : 15-18.

Prasad, R. 1977. *Fertility and Family Planning among Hutment Dwellers of Patna.* Patna University: Demographic Research Center, Patna.

Premrajan, K.C. and Srinivasan D.K. 1994. Child Health Care: Is there a gender difference? *Journal of Family Welfare,* 40(**1**): 7-14.

Purnia, K. and Singh, K. 1984. Prospects of family planning in rural Haryana. *Population Education News,* 11(**1**): 23-28

Rajyalakshmi, C. 1991. Health Modernity in Tribal and Non-Tribal Women in Santhal Pargana. *Social Change,* 21(**1**) : 23-38.

Ramachandran, P. 1983. Interrelationship between breast feeding and weaning practices and mortality - A review. Paper presented at an *ICMR/Ford Foundation Workshop on Child Health, Nurtition and Family Planning,* New Delhi.

Ramachandran, L. and Muthuswamy, P. 1994. *An*

Assessment of Maternal Mortality and its Causes. A Research Report, PRC, Tamil Nadu.

Randhawa, I. And Kanwar, J.S. 1990. An epidemiological study of low birth weigth. *Journal of Obstetrics and Gynaecology of India,* **40**: 60-65.

Ranganathan, H.N. and Rao, V. N.1993. Maternal Health Care: Impact of training supervision and community education. *Journal of Family Welfare,* 39(**2**): 34-37.

Ranjan A. 1998. Maternal Mortality in Madhya Pradesh. *Journal of Family Welfare,* 44(**4**): 55-61.

Rao, D.B. 2000. *The HIV/AIDS and NGO.* Discovery Publishing House, Delhi.

Reddy, S. 1995. Breast feeding-practices, problems and prospects. *Journal of Family Welfare,* 41(**4**): 43-51.

Rohde, J.E. 1992. Strtegies to Sustain immunization coverage in India. *Indian Paediatrics,* 29 (**1**): 15-22.

Russel, R. V. 1975. *Tribes and Castes of the Central Provinces of India.* Vol. II, III & IV, Cosmo Publications, Delhi.

Sahay, M. 1993. Health Status of Tribal in India. *Social Change,* 23(**2&3**): 172-178.

Sahay, M. and Singh, S.K. 1995. Modernity in Tribal Hindus. *Social Change,* 19(**4**): 74-92.

Saxsena, D.N. 1988. *Maternal and Infant Care Practice in Rural Areas of India.* Research Report, Population Research Center, Lucknow.

Sarker, Prafulla. C. 2000 Practice of immunization and its impact on maternal and child health care progress in Bangladesh, challenges for its sustainability. *South Asian Anthropologist,* 21(**2**): 79-84.

Sebastian, E.V. 1972, Integration of Family Planning with Maternal and Child Health, Nutrition and General

Health Services. (In) *International Planned Parenthood Federation*, Indian Ocean Region, Population, Development and the Environment, Report of the Proceedings, Bombay.

Seetalaxmi, A.G. 1969. A study of Intra-spousal communication. Bulletin of the Institute of Rural Health and Family Planning, *Gandhigram*, 4 (**3**): 177-182.

Sengupta, S. and Kumar, A. 1977. Immunization in Maternity Homes: A critical review. Population Centre, Lucknow, IPP, *News Letter*, 5(**3**).

Sengupta, S and Gode, A.G. 1987. The study of maternal morbidity and mortality in a North-Indian hospital, a nine years review. *Journal of Obstetrics and Gynaecology*, **37**: 299-400.

Shariff, A. 1989. Societal determinants of the regional differentials in India's family planning programme performance. *Demography India*, 18(**1&2**):135-140.

Sharma, A.N., Yadav, A. and Jain, A. 2002. *The Sedentrized Lohar Gadiyas of Malthon*. Northern Book Centre, New Delhi.

Sharma, K. 1979. *The Kondha of Orissa*. Concept Publishing Company, New Delhi.

Sharma, V. 1988. *Knowledge, Attitude and Practice: Assessment of Opinion Leaders from Four Tribal Block in Udaipur District With Reference to Health, Sanitation and Family Planning*. Ph.D. Thesis, Sukhadia University, Udaipur. (Unpublished)

Sharma, V. and Sharma, A. 1991. Is the female child being neglected? Immunization in India. *Health Policy and Planning*, 6(**3**): 287-290.

Sharma, V. and Sharma, A. 1992. Health profile of pregnant adolescents among selected tribal population in Rajasthan, India. *Journal of Adolescent Health*, 13(8) : 696-698.

Siddh, K.K. 1974. *Family Planning: Knowledge, Attitude and Practice in Family Planning: the Religious Factor*. Abhinav Publication, New Delhi.

Singh, A.K. 1983. Health Modernity education in India. *Social Change*, 13(2): 27-34.

Singh, A.K., Jaiswal, M. and Choudhari, S. 1996. Reproductive and Child Health Education in two tribal villages. *Social Change*, 26(3&4): 140-147.

Singh, A.K. Jaiswal, M. and Hans, A. 1991. Understanding Health of the Tribals. *Social Change*, 21(1) : 3-22.

Singh, A.K., Jaiswal, M., Hans, A., Arora, A., Choudharyi, A. and Jabbi, M.K. 1987a. Family Planning and Child Care in Rural Tribals of Chotanogpur. *Social Change*, 17(3): 86-95.

Singh, A.K., Sinha, S.K., Singh, S.N., Jaiswal, M. and Jabbi, M.K. 1987b. The Myth of the healthy tribal. *Social Change*, 17(1): 3-23.

Singh, A.K., Sinha, S.K., Singh, S.N., Jaiswal, M. and Jabbi, M.K. 1988. Population - Health Education in the Tribals of South Bihar. *Social Change*, 18(1): 3-29.

Singh, J.P. and Dasgupta, A.1983. Social and culture consideration of sterlization; A case study of Patna. *Demography India*, 12(1): 11-22.

Singhal, D.C. 1992. Maternal and child care in India. *Social Change*, 22(3): 132-145.

Srinivasan, K. and Sugathan, T. N. 1976. *Provision of Maternal and Child Health Services as a Basis of Motivation of Family Planning*: An empirical Investigation Through Record Linkage, Research Report, Population Research Centre, Bangalore.

Srivastava, J.N. and Saxena, D.N. 1988. *Hindu-Muslim Differentials in Family Size Ideals and Contraceptive : Attitude and Practices in Uttar Pradesh.* Research Report, Population Research Centre. Lucknow.

Suman, A.S. and Ansari, G.K. 2001. Reproductive health care of women in rural areas: An exploratory study in Nilgiris district in Tamil Nadu. *Journal of Family Welfare,* 47(**1**): 50-55.

Tandan, R.K. 1999. *Organising Childcare Services,* Rajat Publications, New Delhi.

Tawar, P.P. and Bhatia, P.S. 1985. *Utilization of Health and Family Welfare Services in Rajasthan.* A baseline survey report, NIHFW, New Delhi.

Thimmayamma, B.V.S. and Vidyaviati, M. 1980. Infant feeding practices of working mothers in an urban area. *Indian Journal of Medical Research,* **72**:834-839.

United Nations Children's Fund 1989. *State of World's Children.* Oxford University Press, New Delhi.

United Nations Children's Fund 1991. *Children and Women in India*: a situation analysis. UNICEF, New Delhi.

United Nations Children's Fund 1995. *The Progress in Indian States.* UNICEF, New Delhi.

Varma, N. 2001. Reproductive and sexual health of adolescents: An NGO experience. *Health for the Millions,* 27(**3**): 42-44.

Vijayakumar, S. and Chakrapani, C. 1995. Availability, accessibility and utilization of rural health services. *Journal of Family Welfare,* 41(**3**): 52-60.

Visaria, L. and Visaria P. 1990. Quality of services and family planning in Gujarat state, India: An Exploratory Analysis, Presented at ICOMP International

Conference on the Strategy of Quality Service delivery in Population Programmes, Kaula-lampur, Malaysia.

Vlassoff, C. 1984. A micro- study of culture and fertility in rural Maharashtra. Pater Presented at the *IUSSP Seminar on Micro Approaches to Demographic Research*, Canberra.

Walia, B.N.S., Garmbhir, S.K. and Bhatia, U. 1974. Breast feeding and weaning practices in an urban population. *Indian Pediatrics*, **11**: 133-141.

World Health Organization 1981.*Collaborative Study on Breastfeeding*. A report, WHO, Geneva.

World Health Organization 1991. *Maternal Mortality : A Global Factbook*. World Health Oranisation, Geneva.

Yadav, A., Sharma, A.N. and Jain, A. 2002. Reproductive behaviour among the Sedentrized Lohar Gadiyas of Malthon of Sagar District, Madhya Pradesh. *Vanyajati*, 50(2): 24-27.

Yesudian, C.A.K. 1988. *Utilization of Health Services by the Urban Poor: A Study of the Deonar Maternity Home Health Post Areas*. Survey Report, Tata Institute of Social Sciences. Bombay.

Yesudian, C.A.K. 1989. *Health Services Utilization in Urban India*. Mittal Publication, New Delhi.

Zoe, M. and Mahendra, S. 2001. Antenatal care, care seeking and morbidity in rural Karnataka, India: Results of a prospective study. *Asia-Pacific Population Journal*, 16(2): 11-28.